VACCINE
WHISTLEBLOWER

EXPOSING AUTISM RESEARCH FRAUD AT THE CDC

Kevin Barry, Esq.

Foreword by
Robert F. Kennedy, Jr., JD, LLM

Preface by
Dr. Boyd E. Haley

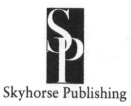

Skyhorse Publishing

For Owen, Griffin, and Isaac.

Copyright © 2015, 2017 by Kevin Barry, Esq.

All rights reserved. No part of this book may be reproduced in any manner without the express written consent of the publisher, except in the case of brief excerpts in critical reviews or articles. All inquiries should be addressed to Skyhorse Publishing, 307 West 36th Street, 11th Floor, New York, NY 10018.

Skyhorse Publishing books may be purchased in bulk at special discounts for sales promotion, corporate gifts, fund-raising, or educational purposes. Special editions can also be created to specifications. For details, contact the Special Sales Department, Skyhorse Publishing, 307 West 36th Street, 11th Floor, New York, NY 10018 or info@skyhorsepublishing.com.

Skyhorse® and Skyhorse Publishing® are registered trademarks of Skyhorse Publishing, Inc.®, a Delaware corporation.

Visit our website at www.skyhorsepublishing.com.

10 9 8 7 6 5 4 3

Library of Congress Cataloging-in-Publication Data is available on file.

Cover design by Erik Nanstiel

ISBN: 978-1-5107-2730-4
Ebook ISBN: 978-1-5107-0638-5

Printed in the United States of America

"Universal Declaration on Bioethics and Human Rights
Article 6—Consent

1. Any preventive, diagnostic and therapeutic medical intervention is only to be carried out with the prior, free and informed consent of the person concerned, based on adequate information. The consent should, where appropriate, be express and may be withdrawn by the person concerned at any time and for any reason without disadvantage or prejudice."

—The United Nations Educational, Scientific and Cultural
Organization (UNESCO), October 2005

CONTENTS

Contents

Preface

Due to my extensive experience in dealing with government agencies regarding issues of mercury and organic mercury toxicities, I was asked to write a preface for this presentation of the recorded conversations between Dr. Brian Hooker (a parent of an autistic child and an activist for autistic children and their parents) and Dr. William W. Thompson (a Senior Scientist with the Center for Disease Control and Prevention, the CDC).

My academic research resulted in my presentation of data on laboratory level thimerosal toxicity at both the 2000 and 2004 Institutes of Medicine meetings regarding vaccine safety. I was exposed to the opinions of both autistic parents and the CDC on the involvement of vaccines, or components of vaccines, in the well-recognized epidemic of autism that started in approximately 1990. I came to this issue as a scientist. I am not the parent of a child with autism, nor, to my knowledge, are any of my relatives afflicted with this illness.

I truly wish I could write that I think vaccines are as safe and effective as the CDC claims they are, but I cannot. I have read hundreds of articles published in scientific journals, both supporting and questioning the safety and the potential toxicity of vaccines, with many describing the basic biochemical and cellular toxic effects of vaccine components such as thimerosal and aluminum. Based on my extensive study of this issue over many years, as I write today, I have sincere and severe doubts about the safety and efficacy of vaccines (both those currently used and those that have been removed from the market) used to inoculate our children against infectious diseases. I am specifically concerned that current supporters of today's vaccine program quote as fact research results in articles proven to be based on manipulated data.

The material herein, mostly presented by Dr. Thompson, a self-described whistleblower, details his experiences with inappropriate CDC handling of data used in peer reviewed journals to demonstrate vaccine safety. His statements are incredibly damaging to the reputation and credence of any work that the CDC supported that addresses the autism and vaccine safety issue. Indeed it implies that the American public cannot trust the health of its children to the most important health regulatory agency within the US government. The inability of the CDC to identify the causes of Autism Spectrum Disorders, no matter the rate, is apparent. Perhaps the reluctance of its leaders to appropriately consider potential causes that they find unpleasant to accept is the reason. Dr. Thompson's stated wish to be subpoenaed by Congress, along with his coworkers involved, gives credence to his statements implying malfeasance within the CDC.

Vaccine safety goes well beyond autism as well. It is disturbing to think that the comparatively high infant mortality rate that the US has compared to its peer nations, many of which have schedules far less aggressive than the US's schedule and many of which do not mandate vaccination, may be explained, at least in part, by the possible illness-inducing effects of our vaccine program. Would the lack of safety research be an explanation for the CDC's claim of one in six children with neurodevelopmental issues in the United States?

This series of conversations between Drs. Hooker and Thompson are gut-wrenching and almost unbelievable to accept, but they are true and accurate. However, with the recent success in the push by the vaccine industry supporters to demand all children be vaccinated, this series is as necessary for parents and pediatricians to read as it is for our congressional members to read and investigate thoroughly.

Dr. Boyd E. Haley
Professor Emeritus and former Chairman of the Department
of Chemistry, University of Kentucky

Foreword

I have always been fiercely pro-vaccine. I had all six of my children vaccinated. I believe that vaccines have saved millions of lives and that broad vaccine coverage is desirable. To achieve those goals, we need safe vaccines, transparent and reliable science, and an independent regulatory agency. The extraordinary revelations in this book by CDC insider and whistleblower Dr. William Thompson prove that, unfortunately, we have none of these.

The continued presence of Thimerosal, a mercury-based preservative, in vaccines is emblematic of the pervasive corruption and mismanagement in the CDC's vaccine program revealed by Dr. Thompson in the pages that follow. For years I have raised concerns about the pharmaceutical industry's persistent use of Thimerosal in vaccines eighteen years after FDA banned the use of this neurotoxin in other medicines and forced its removal from over one thousand over-the-counter drugs. Thimerosal is still present in four American vaccines, including giant "bolus" doses in fifty million flu vaccines administered each year to American adults, pregnant women, and infants. While the industry has removed Thimerosal from pediatric vaccines administered to American children, we still inoculate one hundred million children in developing nations with vaccines containing massive loads of neurotoxic mercury—a course that will come back to haunt our nation in many dreadful ways.

In 2014, I published a book with Dr. Mark Hyman and Dr. Martha Herbert, *Thimerosal: Let the Science Speak*, a complete review of the hundreds of peer-reviewed studies that examine the effects of Thimerosal in animals and humans. Those studies link Thimerosal to a vast inventory of grim neurological disorders now epidemic in children, including ADD, ADHD, speech delay, tics, ASD, and autism. Other studies demonstrate Thimerosal's causation to asthma and a tenfold increase in Alzheimer's in adults exposed to Thimerosal-laced flu shots. During three years of research, we were not able to find a single credible study in the open public health literature that shows Thimerosal to be safe. These impacts are no surprise. Mercury is a potent brain poison hundreds of times more toxic than lead. Science shows that the ethyl mercury in Thimerosal is fifty times as toxic to brain cells and twice as persistent in the brain as the heavily regulated methylmercury in fish. Thimerosal is so toxic that when a doctor carelessly shatters a multidose flu vial, state laws require evacuation of the building and clean-up by trained hazmat crews wearing protective boots, gloves, and respirators. Common sense should tell us that it's not a good idea to inject this poison into infants or expectant mothers. Nevertheless, motivated by greed and bureaucratic self-preservation, the pharmaceutical industry and its captive regulators at the CDC continue to promote Thimerosal as safe.

The debate over Thimerosal and vaccine safety has precipitated a crisis not just in public health but also in journalism. During my ten years observing this debate, I've been puzzled by the baseless insistence by media outfits and reporters that it is somehow safe to inject mercury into humans. The most troubling aspect of this controversy has been a widespread reluctance by journalists to actually read the peer-reviewed science. Reporters simply parrot the talking points of corrupt public health regulators and vaccine industry spokesmen. Instead of arguing the science, they recite the credentials of the CDC's Vaccine Safety Division and repeat the CDC's hollow claim that "The science shows Thimerosal is safe."

With the publication of Kevin Barry's *Vaccine Whistleblower: Exposing Autism Research Fraud at the CDC*, any claims of credibility for the CDC's science has collapsed.

Barry built his book upon four legally taped conversations between CDC senior vaccine safety scientist Dr. William Thompson and Simpson College professor and epidemiologist, Dr. Brian Hooker. Thompson is an author of two of the three epidemiological studies on American populations touted by the CDC to "prove" the safety of Thimerosal. He is also coauthor of the CDC's seminal 2004 study known as DeStefano 2004, which dismissed the link between the MMR vaccine and autism. That study has been cited in ninety-one subsequent published studies and is one of the principal cornerstones for claims by the CDC and the vaccine industry that vaccines do not cause autism. Thompson now confesses that he and his fellow CDC researchers found a strong autism signal in children who received the MMR vaccine before their third birthday. Then, under orders from their bosses and in violation of the study protocols, the scientists eliminated this data from the final published study, in order to fool the public about vaccine safety.

In the pages that follow, you will read Thompson's shocking first-hand description of the pervasive culture of corruption at the CDC's Immunization Safety Office and the techniques employed by the bureaucracy to enforce message discipline and keep doctors and the public in the dark about the dangers of some vaccines. Thompson, who is still employed at the CDC's National Center for Birth Defects and Developmental Disabilities, discloses in sickening details how scientists in the Immunization Safety Office, under order from corrupt bosses, systematically conceal the statistical links between vaccines and brain injuries, particularly autism. Dr. Thompson told Dr. Hooker that whenever the CDC finds an adverse effect from vaccines, the agency supervisors assemble CDC scientists in a room and order them to massage the data until they have devised a gimmick for eliminating the unwanted signal.

"I have a boss who is asking me to lie." Dr. Thompson now confesses, "The higher-ups wanted to do certain things and I went along with it..."

Dr. Thompson is not an insignificant figure at the CDC. He is the author and coauthor of all three of the leading CDC studies that supposedly exonerate vaccines as a causative agent of autism, DeStefano 2004, Thompson 2007, and Price 2010.

In 2008, Dr. Paul Offit, the vaccine industry's foremost spokesman and the pharmaceutical industry's principle advocate for the continued use of mercury in vaccines, praised Dr. Thompson's "wonderful" 2007 study as the "definitive" study proving Thimerosal safety.

In over thirty conversations with Hooker, Thompson disclosed in great detail the CDC's tricks for executing the fraud. "Statistics don't lie," the saying goes, "but statisticians do." Epidemiological or population studies are well-suited to arriving at prearranged results. One could design an epidemiological study to prove that sex does not make you pregnant—just remove all the pregnant people from the pool before you study it! That's the gimmick the CDC has perfected, in order to preserve the illusion of Thimerosal safety. In the 2007 study, CDC scientists removed the low IQ individuals and individuals with autism or other neurological diagnosis from the pool before even beginning their study on Thimerosal exposure. Despite those crooked presentations, scientists still found a persistent signal for tics, a family of grave neurological injuries, including Tourette's syndrome that are associated with autism. Thompson now says that his bosses at the CDC pressured him to also alter the results of that study in order to conceal Thimerosal's risks. Thompson says that the CDC's Developmental Disabilities branch chief, Frank DeStefano, and his superiors at the CDC pressured him to manipulate the study's findings and to bury the truth. In response to this pressure, the published version downplayed data showing that Thimerosal causes "tics."

"Thimerosal from vaccines causes tics." Thompson tells us, "I can say tics are four times more prevalent in kids with autism. There is biologic plausibility right now to say that Thimerosal causes autism-like features."

After concealing these findings in the published version, the CDC aggressively touted Thompson's crooked study to exculpate mercury. That propaganda campaign laid the ground for the CDC's recommendation that Thimerosal-laden flu vaccines be administered to pregnant women despite the fact that the FDA had never approved use of flu vaccines during pregnancy and that Thimerosal is contradicted during pregnancy by the chemical manufacturer's own inserts and its Material Safety Data Sheets. Thompson stated, "Do you think a pregnant mother would want to take a vaccine that they know caused tics? Absolutely not! I would never give my wife a vaccine that I thought caused tics."

The damage isn't isolated to mercury-triggered neurological injuries. When Thompson discovered that the MMR vaccine was causing dramatic rises in autism in African American boys, his CDC bosses ordered him to keep his mouth shut. Thompson coauthored a seminal 2004 study on the MMR subsequently published in *Pediatrics*. He now admits that, under pressure from his superiors, his team fraudulently withheld data demonstrating a 340 percent higher risk of autism in African American boys who received that vaccine on time compared to boys who delayed the vaccine. When Thompson sent a letter complaining about the fraud to CDC director Julie Gerberding, her lackey, Robert Chen, chief at the Immunization Safety branch, stalked Thompson into the CDC's parking lot to menace and threaten him. Thompson would be fired, Chen explained pointedly, if his complaints persisted. For eleven years, the CDC cited the fraudulent DeStefano/Thompson 2004 study to "prove" to journalists and the public that the autism link was disproven. Because of that study, doctors and public health officials continue to give that vaccine to children, even though its links to autism are proven in this and many other studies. On the basis of all the population data and the CDC's most recent autism incidence estimates, at least 100,000 African American male children could have been spared debilitating neurological injury if the CDC scientists had told the truth when Thompson and his team first discovered the increased risk in 2001. You will read Thompson confessing, "I have great shame now when I meet families with kids with autism because I've—I've been part of the problem."

Thompson's shocking confession of lies and scandal verifies the already well-documented corruption at the CDC's Immunization Safety Office. In recent years federal investigators and Congressional committees have issued a series of scathing reports highlighting conflicts of interest at the CDC's vaccine and research divisions. A 2000 report by the Government Reform Committee entitled "Conflicts of Interest in Vaccine Policy Making" identified a long inventory of corrupt financial ties between regulators and vaccine makers in FDA and CDC vaccine programs that are diverting the agency from its task of safeguarding public health. A 2007 US Senate investigation by Senator Tom Coburn, "CDC Off Center," found widespread corruption and mismanagement at the CDC's vaccine programs. In 2008 an investigation by the Office of the Inspector General (IG) of HHS found that 97 percent of special government advisors on committees in the CDC vaccine program failed to disclose necessary information about conflicts of interest (Levinson, 2008). Those findings prompted a series of criminal investigations. In March 2014 the US Office of Research Integrity (ORI) director, David Wright, quit his job and issued a searing letter claiming pervasive scientific misconduct in biomedical research at the CDC, the National Institute of Health (NIH), and the Public Health Service (PHS), all part of HHS, which he characterized as "a remarkably dysfunctional bureaucracy."

Despite such evidence, mainstream journalists continue to revere the CDC as a source of impeccable and unbiased medical information. *Slate*'s Laura Helmuth, vice president of the National Association of Science Writers, recently lambasted Thimerosal critics as "arrogant crackpots." My skepticism about Thimerosal earned me Helmuth's scorn. Helmuth labeled me "a relentless conspiracy theorist." Helmuth assured her readers that CDC employees were "some of the best public servants this country has." Journalists like Helmuth uniformly refuse to report the myriad of problems at the CDC's vaccine program. Adopting the government/industry orthodoxy, they censor vaccine safety advocates who urge the removal of Thimerosal from vaccines.

The pharmaceutical industry spent $3.8 billion in direct marketing to TV, radio, newspapers, and other direct marketing outlets in 2013 and an astonishing $5.4 billion in 2005. Some vaccine safety advocates have questioned whether that cash pipeline accounts, in part, for the mainstream media's blackout of discussions of vaccine safety.

The fraudulent studies that Thompson exposes have oft been cited as the principal proofs of the CDC's claim that vaccines are not linked to the autism epidemic. Thompson's revelation in this book calls into question the validity of the entire body of research that families, medical professionals, and policymakers relied upon in making health decisions for children.

Dr. Thompson invoked the protection of the Federal Whistleblower Statute following the release of portions of the audio of his conversations with Dr. Hooker over the summer of 2014. He issued a statement through his attorney, Rick Morgan of Morgan Verkamp of Cincinnati, Ohio; Dr. Thompson explained that Dr. Hooker had taped the four conversations without permission. However, Thompson courageously reaffirmed the truth of those conversations.

"I regret that my coauthors and I omitted statistically significant information in our 2004 article published in the journal Pediatrics. The omitted data suggested that African American males who received the MMR vaccine before age 36 months were at increased risk for autism. Decisions were made regarding which findings to report after the data were collected, and I believe that the final study protocol was not followed."

Thompson and his attorney have handed over thousands of damning CDC documents to Congressman Bill Posey of Florida in the hope that Congress will subpoena him to testify under oath.

"If forced to testify," Thompson promises, "I'm not going to lie. I basically have stopped lying."

In this book, Dr. William Thompson, a critical player in vaccine safety research, stops lying. Will the media and the government finally have the courage to hear what he is saying and act?

—Robert F. Kennedy, Jr., JD, LLM

Introduction

> *"That's the deal . . ., that's what I keep seeing again and again and again . . . where these senior people [at CDC] just do completely unethical, vile things and no one holds them accountable."*
>
> —Dr. William Thompson to
> Dr. Brian Hooker in a recorded phone call, June 12, 2014

As Dr. William Thompson explains to Dr. Brian Hooker in a series of telephone calls legally recorded in 2014, no one has held the Centers for Disease Control and Prevention (CDC) accountable for wrongdoing that implicates the safety and efficacy of the US vaccine program. The result of this lack of accountability may well be a government-enabled pharmaceutical industry scandal of unprecedented scope.

This book contains transcripts of four telephone calls between Dr. William Thompson, a longtime researcher and Senior Scientist involved in vaccine research at the CDC, and Dr. Brian Hooker, an academic with a strong interest in vaccine safety. Dr. Hooker has a vaccine-injured son with autism.

What Thompson says about the way science is really conducted inside the CDC is alarming. He is not the only person who is talking about the CDC's ethical problems:

"There are four federal studies that have looked at CDC and said the vaccine program at CDC is a cesspool of corruption." —Robert F.

Kennedy Jr. on *Newsmax*, 6/1/15 (http://www.newsmax.com/News-front/RFK-Jr-vaccine-CDC-cesspool/2015/06/01/id/648103/#ix-zz3cbJrItmI)

What you will read are the words of a CDC insider. Dr. Thompson acknowledged that it is his voice on the recordings in a statement released 8/27/14 by his attorney, Rick Morgan of Morgan/Verkamp, one of the nation's leading law practices specializing in whistleblower cases (see below).

STATEMENT OF WILLIAM W. THOMPSON, Ph.D., REGARDING THE 2004 ARTICLE EXAMINING THE POSSIBILITY OF A RELATIONSHIP BETWEEN MMR VACCINE AND AUTISM (August 27, 2014)

My name is William Thompson. I am a Senior Scientist with the Centers for Disease Control and Prevention, where I have worked since 1998.

I regret that my coauthors and I omitted statistically significant information in our 2004 article published in the journal Pediatrics. The omitted data suggested that African American males who received the MMR vaccine before age 36 months were at increased risk for autism. Decisions were made regarding which findings to report after the data were collected, and I believe that the final study protocol was not followed. . . .

I have had many discussions with Dr. Brian Hooker over the last 10 months regarding studies the CDC has carried out regarding vaccines and neurodevelopmental outcomes including autism spectrum disorders. I share his belief that CDC decision-making and analyses should be transparent. I was not, however, aware that he was recording any of our conversations, nor was I given any choice regarding whether my name would be made public or my voice would be put on the Internet. . . .

I am providing information to Congressman William Posey, and of course will continue to cooperate with Congress. I have also offered to assist with reanalysis of the study data or development of further studies. For the time being, however, I am focused on my job and my family.

Reasonable scientists can and do differ in their interpretation of information. I will do everything I can to assist any unbiased and objective scientists inside or outside the CDC to analyze data collected by the CDC or other public organizations for the purpose of understanding whether vaccines are associated with an increased risk of autism. There are still more questions than answers, and I appreciate that so many families are looking for answers from the scientific community.

Omitting data to cover up an undesirable outcome in order to reach a predetermined result is research fraud. Dr. Thompson strongly suggests that the CDC staff involved in vaccine safety studies withheld data to bury a connection between vaccine injury and autism.

If Dr. Thompson is correct, scientific truth was placed second to policy interests. The health of children was compromised to protect the vaccine program. The American public has been lied to and children have been unnecessarily injured due to the corruption at the CDC. The financial cost of this corruption to tax payers is staggering. The human cost is incalculable.

On the call with Dr. Hooker dated May 24, 2014, Dr. Thompson is remorseful about his participation in the studies and actions taken by CDC researchers and wishes he had spoken out earlier.

I have great shame now when I meet families with kids with autism because I have been part of the problem . . . Here's what I shoulder. I shoulder that the CDC has put the [autism/vaccine] research ten years behind. Because the CDC has not been transparent, we've missed ten years of research because the CDC is so paralyzed right now by anything related to autism. They're not doing what they should be doing because they're afraid to look for things that might be associated. So anyway there's still a lot of shame with that.

Dr. Thompson is a coauthor on seminal vaccine safety research papers on the MMR vaccine (Measles, Mumps, and Rubella) and thimerosal, a mercury preservative still used in some flu vaccines, including vaccines which are still given to pregnant women and children. Only one vaccine (MMR) and one component of vaccines (thimerosal) have ever been studied by the CDC in relation to autism risk.

Dr. Thompson was a coauthor on both.

Regarding the MMR paper, Dr. Thompson says in his public statement that he and his coauthors "omitted statistically significant information" which showed an increased risk of autism for African American boys who got the MMR vaccine before age three. The paper, which Dr. Thompson says "did not follow the final study protocol," was published in February 2004. If Dr. Thompson and his coauthors had honestly reported the results, additional research would have been required.

Instead, three months later in May 2004, the Institute of Medicine (IOM) used Dr. Thompson's MMR paper to slam the door on future autism and vaccine research.

Immunization Safety Review: Vaccines and Autism (2004)

"This eighth and final report of the Immunization Safety Review Committee examines the hypothesis that vaccines, specifically the measles-mumps-rubella (MMR) vaccine and thimerosal-containing vaccines, are causally associated with autism. The committee reviewed the extant published and unpublished epidemiological studies regarding causality and studies of potential biologic mechanisms by which these immunizations might cause autism.

The committee concludes that the body of epidemiological evidence favors rejection of a causal relationship between the MMR vaccine and autism. The committee also concludes that the body of epidemiological evidence favors rejection of a causal relationship between thimerosal-containing vaccines and autism. The committee further finds that potential biological mechanisms for vaccine-induced autism that have been generated to date are theoretical only.

The committee does not recommend a policy review of the current schedule and recommendations for the administration of either the MMR vaccine or thimerosal-containing vaccines. The committee recommends a public health response that fully supports an array of vaccine safety activities.

In addition, the committee recommends that available funding for autism research be channeled to the most promising areas (emphasis added). *The committee makes additional recommendations regarding surveillance and epidemiological research, clinical studies, and communication related to these vaccine safety concerns."* (https://www.iom.edu/Reports/2004/Immunization-Safety-Review-Vaccines-and-Autism.aspx)

In May 2014, Dr. Thompson told Dr. Hooker that the CDC had put the research ten years behind. Ten years earlier, in May 2004, the IOM issued its report blocking additional federal research funding for autism and vaccines, stating that "available funding for autism research [should] be channeled into the most promising areas," meaning something other than vaccine research. One year has passed since that phone call. Now the CDC has put the research eleven years behind.

From comments made by IOM staff at a closed-door meeting in 2004, which later became public, the result of the IOM safety report appears to have been predetermined. In transcripts from the beginning of IOM's "Safety Review" the Committee Chair, Dr. Marie McCormick, informed other committee members what was expected. Dr. Kathleen Stratton acknowledged McCormick's statement noting that the IOM was instructed to declare vaccines safe, to not change the vaccine schedule, and to not come down that autism was a true side effect.

"Dr. McCormick: . . . [CDC] wants us to declare, well, these things are pretty safe on a population basis (p. 33).

Dr. Stratton: . . . The point of no return, the line we will not cross in public policy is pull the vaccine, change the schedule. We could say it is time to revisit this, but we would never recommend that level. Even recommending research is recommendations for policy. We wouldn't say compensate, we wouldn't say pull the vaccine, we wouldn't say stop the program. (p. 74)

Dr. McCormick: . . . we are not ever going to come down that [autism] is a true side effect . . . (p. 97)" IOM Committee Meeting, 1/12/2001 Closed-Door Meeting Transcript (http://www.putchildrenfirst.org/chapter6.html)

The statistically significant data, which Dr. Thompson and his coauthors did not report, did not fit with the CDC and IOM's predetermined result that autism was not a true side effect of vaccination. The authors found a way to alter the study protocol to fit the predetermined result.

Dr. Thompson's revelations about dishonest vaccine safety research to Dr. Hooker are critically important to policymakers, pediatricians, and parents.

Tens of thousands of parents have reported that their children regressed into autism after adverse vaccine reactions. Parents are forced to rely on the honesty of the CDC about vaccine safety when deciding how to vaccinate their children. Pediatricians are forced to rely on the honesty of the CDC about vaccine safety in deciding how to treat their patients. Policy makers are forced to rely on the honesty of the CDC about vaccine safety when deciding whether to mandate vaccines.

Based on the words of Dr. William Thompson, the CDC has lied to everyone involved in administering and receiving vaccinations.

Dr. Thompson now says "there are more questions than answers" about "whether vaccines are associated with an increased risk of autism." Given Dr. Thompson's revelations, no state legislature should pass another vaccine mandate bill, and no governor should sign one until these questions are answered. No state legislature should pass a bill that removes vaccine exemptions or restricts a person's right to decide what vaccines to take or allow children to receive. Any governor who receives such a bill should refuse his or her signature. Elected officials should call on the President and Congress to take action to protect the safety of children.

Dr. Thompson describes a culture of corruption within the CDC regarding vaccine safety research, which should give pause to any elected official who has placed blind trust in the CDC.

Dr. Hooker legally recorded four calls with Dr. Thompson in 2014. The calls occurred on May 8, May 24, June 12, and July 28. With this excerpt from Dr. Thompson's statement, he verifies that it is his voice on the recordings:

I have had many discussions with Dr. Brian Hooker over the last 10 months regarding studies the CDC has carried out regarding vaccines and neurodevelopmental outcomes including autism spectrum disorders. I share his belief that CDC decision-making and analyses should be transparent. I was not, however, aware that he was recording any of our conversations, nor was I given any choice regarding whether my name would be made public or my voice would be put on the Internet.

What you are about to read are the true words of Dr. Thompson, the Vaccine Whistleblower.

Chapter 1
Executive Summary
of the Four Calls

"The great enemy of the truth is very often not the lie, deliberate, contrived and dishonest, but the myth, persistent, persuasive and unrealistic."

—John F. Kennedy

At a town hall meeting in Los Angeles on June 17, 2015, Dr. Brian Hooker revealed that he and Dr. Thompson had spoken on the phone over thirty times. Dr. Hooker legally recorded four of those calls.

". . . Over the period of November 2013 to August 2014, I had over thirty separate phone conversations with Dr. Thompson. He initially reached out to me in an unsolicited phone conversation to my cell phone. Dr. Thompson and I had talked on the phone and exchanged email correspondences much earlier, between 2002 and 2004, back when I was trying to advise the CDC on their vaccine safety studies related to childhood neurodevelopmental disorders. However, the CDC curtailed my conversations with him in 2004 due to my family's participation in the National Vaccine Injury Compensation Program where we were seeking remuneration for my

own son's vaccine injuries. The phone calls from November 2013 to August 2014 were secret and Thompson did not let CDC officials know that he and I were talking as that could have cost him his employment.

I made the decision to record four of the last phone conversations I had with Dr. Thompson, without his knowledge, based on the revelation of harm to children, caused by the CDC's very dysfunctional and even criminal vaccine safety program. These recordings were obtained legally and involved advice from legal counsel in each instance. . . ."

(http://www.ageofautism.com/2015/06/the-battle-for-california-part-4-the-nation-of-islam-and-the-church-of-scientology-join-the-fight-ag.html)

Call 1—Highlights of the May 8, 2014, call

1. Dr. Thompson wants to "stop lying" about omitting significant data which suggested an elevated risk of autism in a subpopulation (African American males) from a 2004 MMR paper he coauthored.

2. Dr. Thompson says "thimerosal causes tics," thimerosal-containing vaccines "should never be given to pregnant women," and that he would never give a thimerosal-containing vaccine to his own wife. Flu shots with thimerosal are on the recommended vaccine schedule for children, pregnant women, and adults.

3. Dr. Thompson describes how the CDC stonewalls Congressional requests for documents and how the CDC stonewalls requests for information under the Freedom of Information Act.

4. Dr. Thompson says how the CDC and media "love" to "hype" measles and polio outbreaks in order to "scare" the public. In May 2014, Thompson essentially predicted how the CDC and media reacted to the measles outbreak at Disneyland in late 2014.

5. Dr. Thompson says autism research is a "political hot potato" inside the CDC.

6. Dr. Thompson discusses in May 2014, some seven months before the CDC, drug companies, and the press fanned the fires of measles hysteria, that they love to hype and scare people: "But I also have to say these drug companies and their promoters, they're making such a big deal of these measles outbreaks and they now they're making a big deal that polio is coming back and polio comes back all the time in third world countries. It's like a never-ending thing where the press loves to hype it and it scares people."

Call 2—Highlights of the May 24, 2014, call

1. Dr. Thompson says what the CDC has been denying for years: "There is biologic plausibility right now, I really do believe there is, to say that thimerosal causes autism-like symptoms."

2. Dr. Thompson hired a whistleblower attorney in May 2014 to protect his position as an employee at the CDC during the period he hopes to testify before Congress.

3. Dr. Thompson says the CDC is currently sitting on a treasure trove of data pertaining to 1,200 children with autism—including vaccine records of children and their mothers (Rhogam, flu shots). It's called the SEED (Study to Explore Early Development) study.

4. Dr. Thompson says that researchers at the CDC are not looking at the vaccine data, and Dr. Thompson urges that the data be looked at by genuinely independent researchers. Dr. Thompson's suggestion disqualifies CDC partner organizations like Autism Speaks. The founding of Autism Speaks in 2005 was underwritten by a $25 million dollar gift from Home Depot cofounder and billionaire Bernie Marcus. Mr. Marcus is Chairman Emeritus of the CDC Foundation. (More on Autism Speaks in Chapter 9.)

5. Dr. Thompson says CDC staffers Dr. Boyle and Dr. Yeargin-Allsopp were invited to testify at the Congressional hearing

held on May 20, 2014, but they declined the invitation. Thompson says Dr. Yeargin-Allsopp said she "won't" testify and Dr. Boyle said she would "never" testify before Congress again. Knowing this, one can hope Congress will not hesitate to use subpoena power to compel these federal employees to be accountable.

6. Dr. Thompson says the "CDC has put the research ten years behind." Dr. Thompson's MMR paper was published in 2004. The Verstraeten and Madsen papers were published in 2003. The signals on the possible connection between vaccination and autism and other adverse events like tics and verbal IQ were not accurately reported by researchers. Because the CDC researchers omitted significant data, the flow of research was diverted away from vaccination. The autism rate has increased from 1 in 166 in 2004 to 1 in 68 in 2014.

7. Dr. Thompson says "I am part of the problem," and confides that he has "great regret."

8. Dr. Thompson predicts his coauthors at the CDC will try to undermine him when news of his whistleblowing gets out. Dr. Thompson predicts they will argue that he is mentally ill. Fortunately, Dr. Thompson kept his records from the study in question and he has turned those records over to Congress.

Call 3—Highlights of the June 12, 2014, call

1. Dr. Thompson acknowledges that he and his coauthors changed the criteria of their 2004 MMR paper to alter the data in a way which eliminated a signal which indicated that, for African American boys, getting the MMR vaccine "on time" (before age three) increased the risk of an autism diagnosis.

2. Dr. Thompson reveals that because there was no outside review panel on the 2004 MMR paper, there was no one to stop them from changing the criteria.

3. Dr. Thompson describes the difficulty in getting significant findings about adverse health outcomes caused by vaccination published by medical journals.

4. Dr. Thompson reveals that indicted fugitive Dr. Poul Thorsen, who is alleged to have stolen more than $1 million from the CDC, is the purported boyfriend of former CDC researcher Dr. Diana Schendel. Dr. Thorsen has been under indictment since 2011 for stealing more than $1 million dollars for his own personal gain from the CDC by falsifying invoices. According to the indictment, he executed a scheme to defraud and divert this money from approximately February 2004 to February 2010. The missing $1 million CDC grant money flowed through Aarhus University and Odense University Hospital in Denmark. Apparently, Dr. Thorsen and Dr. Schendel have been dating the entire time Dr. Thorsen has been under indictment. Dr. Schendel worked at the CDC from 1993 to 2013. Thompson says she spent the summer of 2003 "in Denmark money laundering with her boyfriend." Dr. Schendel relocated to Denmark after leaving the CDC and currently is employed at Aarhus University. (https:// oig.hhs.gov/fraud/fugitives/profiles.asp)

5. Dr. Thompson says those inside CDC want to include Dr. Schendel in research opportunities going forward with the SEED data. If Dr. Schendel and Dr. Thorsen are actually a couple, one can hope the CDC will not employ Dr. Schendel while her partner is still a fugitive indicted felon.

6. Dr. Thompson describes former CDC director Julie Gerberding taking a job as President of Merck Vaccines as "dark." Like many parents, Dr. Thompson appears to share the opinion that Dr. Gerberding's choosing to work for a corporation which she used to regulate was shady, dirty, or "dark." The MMR vaccine is manufactured by Merck. Dr. Gerberding was the head of the CDC in the early 2000 when the studies alleging the safety of the MMR vaccine were done. Just after the required waiting period of

a year and a day of leaving the CDC, Dr. Gerberding took her new position at Merck. She currently is Executive Vice President for Strategic Communications, Global Public Policy and Population Health at Merck, as of December 2014. Dr. Gerberding is one of many researchers using the revolving door between government and industry. She has made millions of dollars with Merck and from Merck stocks since leaving the CDC.

7. Dr. Thompson describes a culture at CDC where "senior peo-ple do completely unethical, vile things" and they are "not held accountable." One can hope Congress will hold hearings in the near future to hold them accountable. Hopefully, someday we will also have a president willing to hold the CDC accountable.

8. Dr. Thompson makes an excellent policy recommendation regarding the CDC and the future of vaccine safety. Dr. Thompson suggests moving vaccine safety out of the CDC. He suggests a structure similar to the Federal Aviation Administration (FAA) and the National Transportation Safety Board (NTSB). With this change, the CDC can concentrate on vaccine promotion while a separate agency would be responsible for vaccine safety.

Call 4—Highlights of the July 28, 2014, call

1. Dr. Thompson describes how CDC whitewashes and waters down attempts to replicate adverse effects from previous vaccine safety research. Data showing negative health effects from vaccination would sometimes "disappear" between submission of an original manuscript to a peer-reviewed journal and publication.

2. Dr. Thompson says there is a "very biased political agenda" inside the CDC. One way CDC blocks future vaccine safety research funding is to give research on this issue a "low-priority score" so those projects will lose out to other projects in funding competition.

3. Dr. Thompson speculates that the Verstraeten study (2003) may have EXCLUDED specialty clinics from the data in order to game the data, in a reverse way that the Madsen Denmark paper

INCLUDED specialty clinics to game the data. According to Dr. Thompson, when researchers "don't like what they are finding" in the data, they "adjust" it.

4. Dr. Thompson tells Dr. Hooker that he provided Representative Darrell Issa and Representative Bill Posey with 100,000 documents regarding vaccine safety research, which would assist a Congressional investigation, some of which Dr. Hooker has had a chance to review inside Congressional offices.

Chapter 2
Call 1

First call: May 8, 2014
Thompson: "I have basically stopped lying."

On May 8, 2014, Dr. Brian Hooker called Dr. William Thompson to discuss vaccine research at the CDC. This was the first of four recorded calls they would have over the next several weeks.

****

DR. THOMPSON: Brian?

DR. HOOKER: How are you?

DR. THOMPSON: Alright, how you doin'?

DR. HOOKER: [*laughing*] Oh, I don't know. I've been better, um, I don't know, uh, sometimes I have, I get a little depressed by all the stuff and it gets to me after a while. I'm just having one of those days, ya know, but, uh . . . So, how are things going? Are you, are, are, I would imagine you've still got kids in school, my son's home schooled so it doesn't really matter. When we take vacation, we just decided we're gonna take vacation. I'm off for the school year. We've had our final exams and everything. So I'm just focusing in on um ya know some of the research I'm doing.

I emailed you um a while back about, I just wanted to get your thoughts on ya know and ideas if you would have any ideas on how to fix this. I mean, how, how would, if you were in a position to do so, how would we ban [mercury in vaccines]. Ya know first and foremost I think getting thimerosal out of vaccines is just long overdue and . . .

DR. THOMPSON: Let me tell you my thought on that, okay? So, in the United States the only vaccine [flu shot] it is still in is for pregnant women right? So, my theory on that, is that the drug companies think that if it is in at least that one vaccine then no one could argue that it should be out of the other vaccines outside of the US.

DR. HOOKER: Right.

DR. THOMPSON: So I don't know why they still give it to pregnant women, like that's the last person I would give mercury to.

DR. HOOKER: Yeah, yeah, it makes absolutely no sense. And it's a full 25 micrograms of mercury. In the infants' formulation for the flu shot, ya know, you're not supposed to give flu shots until six months of age. The infants' formulation has 12.5. But, the maternal flu shot still has 25 micrograms and you can give it in any trimester.

DR. THOMPSON: Right. So, I still think, I don't know, I guess you didn't like the idea. I still think that starting a campaign that thimerosal from vaccines cause tics. You start a campaign. You just make that your mantra. I really do believe.

DR. HOOKER: I do like that idea. It does cause tics. The thing that is getting a little disconcerting is that I, ya know, I work with Focus Autism. I work with the head of Focus Autism, a guy named Barry Segal. His wealth came from a roofing company, a roofing materials company called Bradco and he recently wrote a letter to Thomas Frieden. And I wrote the letter. One of the things we highlighted is that even the CDC's publications, there hasn't yet been a publication, except for Tozzi in 2009, you haven't been able to obviate the relationship between thimerosal and tics and tics in boys. And so we get a letter back from Beth Bell. Do you know who she is?

DR. THOMPSON: Yep, I know who she is [*laughing*]. She knows who I am. We know each other.

DR. HOOKER: [*laughing*] And it was like she didn't even read our letter. And she quoted the 2011 Institute of Medicine Vaccine Adverse Events Meeting and Report and the 2011 IOM didn't even consider thimerosal. They were basically told by the CDC not to look at mercury. It wasn't a part of their purview.

DR. THOMPSON: It was supposed to be, they were working on the NVPO [National Vaccine Program Office] plan for a long time and that was being run by Larry Pickering. Larry Pickering ran the, ya know, NVPO plan and I thought, I helped them write that, I thought that they um kept verbal IQ and tics in there. The last time I had looked at it I thought it was in there.

DR. HOOKER: What they did and I have a taped transcript of this. Ellen Clayton who was the chair for the Vaccine Adverse Events and Causality Committee said specifically, "We were not asked to look at mercury at all so we didn't," and this was at, I guess, the petitioners in the National Vaccine Injury Compensation Program have a yearly conference and this particular year it was back in Oakland [California]. And, um, and so they had specific presentations, you were able to get transcripts of the presentations and I did. I got an mp3 of it and I have it on transcript that she . . . So anyhow, what we're doin' is we're gonna go back and um I wrote a rebuttal to the letter that Beth Bell sent. Because it just, there were a lot of things in there that were, it was like.

DR. THOMPSON: Let me just tell you why Beth Bell wrote you. Do you know why she wrote you? Do you understand the structure?

DR. HOOKER: A little bit but go ahead and tell me anyway.

DR. THOMPSON: Alright, they move to quote-unquote make immunization safety independent of the immunization program, they moved it into a separate center. And um so they . . .

DR. HOOKER: She's National Center of Emerging and Zoonotic Infectious Diseases, is that right?

DR. THOMPSON: So it's in a really silly place. They did it theoretically because they were trying to make them independent groups. But they are not independent at all. But um so, that's the bottom line so. She is tight with all these people.

DR. HOOKER: Oh, absolutely. I have no doubt. But where do we push? One of the things that I . . .

DR. THOMPSON: Here's what I . . . Let me just say . . . I see a lot of your stuff online. I saw that you interviewed Congressman Posey, is it?

DR. HOOKER: That was not my best interview. I basically was the king of "um" [laughing] I was also breathing heavily in the phone. I did not do a good job.

DR. THOMPSON: I just think there has to be a mantra. The mantra should be, "We know thimerosal causes tics." That's been demonstrated. That's been demonstrated in the big studies. And just keep saying that, "We know thimerosal causes tics." 'Cause the CDC never said that thimerosal doesn't cause tics. The CDC always says thimerosal doesn't cause autism. You have to take it off that. You have to take it off that. And I really do think it's a public relations campaign. But I also have to say these drug companies and their promoters, they're making such a big deal of these measles outbreaks and they are now, they're making a big deal that polio is coming back and polio comes back all the time in third world countries. It's like a never-ending thing where the press loves to hype it and it scares people. It scares the crap out of people when they hype those two types of outbreaks. I think as they teach you at the CDC, you have to stay on message. And the message I think to start getting out and then you wouldn't have the press jumping on you saying, "Well vaccines don't cause autism." If you said, "Yeah, that's true, but vaccines do cause tics." And then eventually, eventually you could get the message over to oh tics are like five times as common among kids with autism.

DR. HOOKER: Right, it's about four times, but, yes, absolutely.

DR. THOMPSON: I do think that it's staying on message with something different than autism because the press and everyone, you know, Jenny McCarthy, all those people. You bring up autism and vaccines you just get hammered. Who's the company that, who sponsored one of your groups?

DR. HOOKER: Oh, Chili's.

DR. THOMPSON: Yeah, Chili's just got fried. They just completely got fried.

DR. HOOKER: Yeah, I saw that, yeah.

DR. THOMPSON: So I think in the short term, you take it off to something that's true and it's a different story, it's a different story. And you can point to that Italy study (Tozzi et al. 2009) and just look at the means and the means are quite different in that study for tics. I really do think that study actually supports the idea. And then the other thing about the Italy study, the Italy study was the only randomly assigned study and it was a much smaller exposure so if you find something in there and they found two positive effects, right, if I'm recalling correctly, so again, ya know, a study that is randomly assigned, it's the only study I know where there was random assignment and you found two negative associations where it was increased likelihood of maternal, I mean, verbal IQ and I can't remember the other one. But tics, I'm telling you, if my recollection is correct, tics were significant in earlier drafts of the paper.

DR. HOOKER: And what happened with that information request? They put it into the FOIA office and . . .

DR. THOMPSON: You know, and once it's in the FOIA office, it's gone.

DR. HOOKER: It's gonna take forever.

DR. THOMPSON: It's going to take two or three years, right. They tell me, they're two and a half years behind, and they actually said with Posey thing treat it as a FOIA because he's not the head of a committee. So, I just, again, you gotta come up with a different message where you won't get hammered and they can't deny it. Right? The only thing I know for sure, is that I can say that pretty confidently, vaccines cause tics. We replicated that. The Barile article replicated that and showed that once you took into account the number of tests and reduced them down to constructs, the one thing you couldn't get to go away was the tic effect.

DR. HOOKER: Was the tic effect, right. I agree. And I'm even using that in my son's vaccine court case, because he has tics and so, we have that. It's been confirmed in several studies, not to mention your study and then the Barile study that was the reanalysis from 2012. And I'll go back and look at those means on Tozzi as well.

DR. THOMPSON: Look at the means. Look at the means, they're very close. You could do a simple t-test and see they're very close to significance. The other thing I wanted to ask you. Have you ever contacted Dr. Dorea in South America, the person who has done the vaccine studies?

DR. HOOKER: Yeah, I'm in contact with Jose. I'm in contact with Jose.

DR. THOMPSON: Is it a male or a female?

DR. HOOKER: It's a male. And then I believe the way that it goes is that his wife works with him as well. So there's a male and a female.

DR. THOMPSON: So they're the two scientists who actually seem motivated and seem to try wanting to study the problem. I don't know if they still are, but . . .

DR. HOOKER: I will . . . You make a good point and because I'm looking at other scientists who do not have quote-unquote tarnished reputations to um to look at these, to look at the work I'm doing right and because it doesn't really do me any favors to publish with the Geiers. I mean, they're good friends. I've been friends with them for over ten years now. But, I'm not doing myself any favors.

DR. THOMPSON: No, it would be like publishing with Jenny McCarthy. Anything that has their name on it people immediately dismiss. The other thing for you to consider is to find a couple of scientists you trust and to have them publish your results. Don't put yourself as an author.

DR. HOOKER: You know, I'm not very high on the list myself.

DR. THOMPSON: I know, I know, I'm just saying [*laughing*], use a pseudonym. I wouldn't do that. But I'm just saying but if you're really serious about this. You find a couple of good scientists, you walk them through what you're doing, if you can convince a couple of good scientists that what you're doing makes sense and then you encourage them to submit papers. And here is the other thing, is you gotta get it out of the medical journals, you gotta move it to the psychology journals. I don't know if you saw but the Barile article got published in a psychology journal. It wasn't actually, it was like Pediatric Psychology.

DR. HOOKER: It was the Journal of Pediatric Psychology, I saw that.

DR. THOMPSON: Right, but if you get it out of the medical world and into the psychology world, you are not going to get as much bias from the medical establishment that has such a strong hold over these medical journals.

DR. HOOKER: Yeah, that makes a lot of sense. I'm not as well traveled in that realm. Is the Journal of Pediatric Psychology a good one to look at?

DR. THOMPSON: It's a great journal. It is a very good journal. We got great reviews from that journal. I'll tell you. They actually made us [unintelligible] our discussion. They actually said, why are you downplaying the association with tics? So, actually made [UI] . . .

DR. HOOKER: [*laughing*] See, this is the deal though. You are a straight shooter. When you did the 2007 paper and the 2012 follow-up paper, you called a spade a spade with the particular effects. This is why when I look at Stehr-Green. Stehr-Green was . . .

DR. THOMPSON: If I could tell you stories about that guy. He just seemed like a used car salesman. It was really frightening to have him doing what he was doing.

DR. HOOKER: Well wasn't he like a . . . was he a park ranger or a forest ranger at the time?

DR. THOMPSON: Yes, I told you about that. He was like a park ranger at the time. He was one of Roger Bernier's former graduate students.

DR. HOOKER: And one of the things I found out, now, just to ask you the question and to let you know I did go to the office of Oversight and Government Reform, Issa's office. I saw what had been turned over. I will say that over 50 percent of it came from you because I can tell what comes from you [*Thompson laughing*]. So over 50 percent of it, in fact, all I did was I got up to the Cs, the letter C in the alphabet for your stuff that was it. The rest of it is still being reviewed by the office of the general counsel somewhere. So I only got up to the letter C on your deck, um . . . There was a lot of stuff, now, um . . . I got kinda worried when I saw that and I believe I know what is going on but I saw that email that you forwarded that office of general counsel is trying to pull together how much effort they've had to put on my FOIAs. That didn't put me in my happy place. Do you think they're just using that to go back to Issa's staff? [pause] Are you still there?

DR. THOMPSON: Yeah, can you hear me?

DR. HOOKER: Yeah, I can, yeah, yeah.

DR. THOMPSON: So here's what happened. I actually talked to my therapist about it on Wednesday. I said I was really tempted to reply to that email. He now knows you by name. I referred to you as Brian. I said I was tempted to reply back to the email and say Elizabeth, ya know, I'd really love to talk to someone in the OGC who wants me to do this cuz I need more guidance, just to find out which lawyer is doing this.

DR. HOOKER: I'm afraid of those people. I'm afraid of Kevin Malone. I'm afraid of Deborah Tress, I mean, these people, ya know, they don't like me.

DR. THOMPSON: They're scumbags. But here's the deal. She is like a twenty-five-year-old and I apologize as I am saying this, she's like a twenty-five-year-old bimbo that they have do their dirty work. So her sending this email, the fact that they didn't come from someone with a lawyer. It came from this woman who's just out of school and just doesn't know her head from her ass. This is the type of stuff they do. They don't say who it's from, they just say OGC.

DR. HOOKER: I don't think that's in my FOIA case. In my FOIA case, there aren't any pending motions. The FOIA appeal right now, the decision basically comes from the appellate judge and so we're . . . both sides have presented their arguments and the appellate judge may come back and ask for more information. So I don't think that has anything to do with the appeals case. I think it has to do with OGC does not want Issa's office to release any of those documents to me. I've seen them. They would not let me take them out of their office and I didn't. Believe you, I was tempted, I had like a half-a-gigabyte hard drive in my pocket that I could have whipped out when nobody was looking and I didn't even use it. I didn't. I don't want to go to Federal prison and so.

DR. THOMPSON: No, you don't.

DR. HOOKER: No. But, this whole thing was very interesting but I do think it has something to do with what's going on with Issa's, ya know, with that information request, so . . .

DR. THOMPSON: I know. I think they want you as far away from those documents as possible.

DR. HOOKER: Right. I mean there were some very compelling things in there and it will be interesting to see what happens, ya know, we'll see. But, I did want to ask, um . . . I pretty much completed the reanalysis on the Destefano MMR study and those spreadsheets that you sent.

DR. THOMPSON: [to someone not on the phone] Yeah, I'm out here talking . . . [to Hooker] What was that?

DR. HOOKER: The spreadsheets that you sent me, race1, race2, and race3. Can I ask where those came from? Were those just ones that you had or where you compiled results or?

DR. THOMPSON: Those were analyses I ran for a group. Every single Excel spreadsheet you've seen was an analysis I ran for our group over a several-year period where I was presenting results to the group.

DR. HOOKER: Right, right, now in, so, so, these were your analysis files and you basically presented them to the group.

DR. THOMPSON: I would on a weekly basis meet with the four coauthors [Destefano, Boyle, Yeargin-Allsopp, and Bhasin] and we would discuss results and you can see how those progressed over time. You want to know the only way I was able to keep track of the dates on those files? The servers would change all the time and they would change the dates on the files so thank goodness I put the actual date in the name of the file because otherwise you wouldn't know the actual date that I had done it. What was that? I was just talking to your daughter.

DR. HOOKER: No, that's fine. That's fine. But the question I had, if you go to race3, then, you had alternative models. You have a results tab. It's like the second tab in the spreadsheet and it looks like on black on-time and the reason why I'm asking this is it's like cuz like I told you before, I got a really strong effect with African American males. And I saw an effect. It was statistically significant at thirty-six months as well as twenty-four months. Wasn't as high at twenty-four obviously, it was like 1.73 or something. So black on-time, was this just a conditional logistic regression that was matched?

DR. THOMPSON: Yeah, yeah, it was a conditional logistic regression.

DR. HOOKER: Okay, the numbers then would, see the way I understand this the odds ratios that you came up with then, if you just ran it as on time then you would get a specific odds ratio but would that be assigned to thirty-six months or how would that work?

DR. THOMPSON: No, on time would be, if I remember it correctly and I don't have it sitting in front of me, but on time would have been that they would have been vaccinated by twenty-four months of age, right? They would have been vaccinated by the recommended age.

DR. HOOKER: Right, by the recommended age. And then it looks like you did this unmatched and then probably also conditional logistic regression and it went up by just a little. They were basically the same. They're basically the same in each one.

DR. THOMPSON: Yep.

DR. HOOKER: So, um, did you ever slice that further just to look at African American males?

DR. THOMPSON: My guess is that I did but I can't tell. Honestly, the only thing in terms of memory, like I can look at those files and I know I ran those things. But I don't know what else I ran, I could look, I could look at the SAS programs, I never looked through those historically but I believe I have them historically. I think they're in, well, I think they're there. I can't remember off the top of my head. Honestly, the way I remember things is I put them into files, I save them, and I go back and review them.

DR. HOOKER: Would you be able to do that? I mean, I . . .

DR. THOMPSON: Yeah, I could tell you, I can send you some of the SAS programs.

DR. HOOKER: Okay, and one of the things I did find in this weird um, when I use the thirty-six-month cut-off for African American males, I only had seven cases in the after thirty-six months. Okay, so the cohort was getting small. So, I had like seven cases and I can't remember how many controls. Obviously, the lion's share of the cases were for individuals who got the MMR before thirty-six months. Now I, when I, I wanted to correct for low birthweight. So I threw out low birthweight. But what I found was that in my cases after, in the cases of individuals that got the MMR after thirty-six months, I wasn't throwing out low birthweight, I was throwing out individuals that didn't have birthweight reported at all. So you basically look at that and it is essentially saying it is the birth certificate cohort. Does that make sense? Let me, I can explain it one other way. When you look at the data and you look at African American male cases of autism, there are seven cases. There are four cases that did have a birth certificate and were normal birth weight and the remaining three cases didn't have a birth certificate so they didn't have birth weight at all.

DR. THOMPSON: That were vaccinated late.

DR. HOOKER: That were vaccinated late and so I did not include that in my analysis because I felt like a cohort, if it had less than five cases in it, I just didn't want to include it.

DR. THOMPSON: Yeah, you're going to be criticized if you did because of that small of a group.

DR. HOOKER: So I threw that particular one out. Don't take this as a criticism, I'm just trying to understand what was in the paper.

DR. THOMPSON: Let me just clarify to you. You can criticize the hell out of this, I don't think it was perfect and I will tell you we were locked in to analyses, that's the problem with all of this. We agreed upfront, actually with this paper we deviated from what we agreed to upfront. So criticize away.

DR. HOOKER: But the only thing, if you look at the final paper, when they looked at the effect of race, they only looked at the birth certificate cohort.

DR. HOOKER: That doesn't seem right to me. Why, you don't need a birth certificate, you don't need a birth certificate . . .

DR. THOMPSON: I agree, I know, I saw you found that immediately. You told me you found that immediately.

DR. HOOKER: Yes, I did find that immediately but I wasn't sure. You know, I want to go back to these things. Bill, I am not an epidemiologist by training.

DR. THOMPSON: No, no, no . . . I just wanted to say, you found what I considered the biggest problem. Here's what I want to be careful of, okay? I want to be careful of not, uh . . . Here's what I want to tell you . . . If I were forced to testify or something like that, I'm not gonna lie, but I also don't want to say things to you right now, that aren't, that aren't in some written form. I want to be very careful about that. I will say if I'm forced, if it comes through some legitimate channels, if I'm forced to answer questions, I'm not going to lie. I basically have stopped lying.

DR. HOOKER: Did you raise that, did you raise that issue at the time?

DR. THOMPSON: I will say I raised this issue. [Edited due to sensitive personal information.]

DR. HOOKER: Good, good, good. I'm glad to hear that. Let me . . . I've jotted down a few notes on this, um . . . One of things I've noticed when I've been back at DC, going through the documents at OGR and you've told this to me several times. Nobody [who works for CDC] is stupid enough to put in an email, "Let's dilute down this relationship." Or get rid of this relationship.

DR. THOMPSON: Never, never, never, never.

DR. HOOKER: But what is said in these closed-door meetings? Do people say, "Oh this is unacceptable" or do they just say, "Oh this can't be right"? Or . . .

DR. THOMPSON: [*laughing*] I wish I could tell you the quote that was said but there is a specific quote about this very finding that will be etched in my head for life.

DR. HOOKER: Okay, you don't have to tell me it. That's fine.

DR. THOMPSON: I'm not going to tell you it. It was by one of the other coauthors. It is etched in my head for life.

DR. HOOKER: Well, you've given me a lot to think about, you always give me a lot to think about. I want to go back and I want to think about this whole issue with tics. If I was to press the soft spot on the CDC in terms of like submitting the response letter, I think the response letter will come back and I'm going to sign this and get some other scientists to sign off on the letter as well as Barry Segal. And one of the things that I've thought regarding thimerosal is that it should go to [current head of the CDC] Frieden because Frieden could be the guy to save the day. I mean, he's got clean hands. I think?

DR. THOMPSON: He does have clean hands. But I don't know where he stands on all of this. I really don't. I do think this. I do think Frieden, I think he has closed himself off from all of this and avoids this and says this is Coleen Boyle and uh Melinda Wharton's problem. I'm guessing, I don't know that for sure. I'm guessing that, right, that this is just a political hot potato. They made a lot of mistakes and there's a lot of documents that they don't want you to see. What I was relieved about when I sent you was what the NCIRD did with the request. They don't usually include you know Melinda Wharton and Kristin Pope in those requests. They usually just include David Shay and I. So we're often the targets of all the FOIAs and they don't make it broader. What I find even funnier is Kristin Pope is the person directing this document gathering.

DR. HOOKER: How odd . . . How odd . . .

DR. THOMPSON: She was thick and deep into all of this. She was the go between. All of the communication went from me to Brooke Barry to Kristin. So everything was filtered through Kristin. And Kristin reports to Melinda Wharton. And it's still the case. It's still . . .

DR. HOOKER: It wasn't really Kristin. Brooke was the one that could not stand me. Brooke Barry could not stand me. I would get on the phone with her and for the longest time I was dealing with Lorine Spencer. And bless her heart, she did the best she could possibly do. And, I was not a nice person, I was very angry, I was a very, very angry person when I was dealing with Lorine Spencer. It is interesting that Kristin is still in the middle of that because when things got switched around I was dealing with Kristin Pope and Brooke Barry.

DR. THOMPSON: Yeah, and I have to tell you. Kristin and Brooke knew I was sitting on a lot of documents. And when I shared all of these documents, Brooke Barry was probably, I mean, you saw my email. She's probably the only person I trusted to give me a straight answer. I went over to her office and I said, "I hear they want us to share everything," and she said, "Yep, they want us to share everything." So, it was the first time they said they wanted anything that was associated with thimerosal.

DR. HOOKER: But they are arm-wrestling with Oversight and Government Reform right now. Big time. I've gone back and forth, I get calls from Oversight and Government Reform staff and they'll have questions for me. They want to know about the litigation because CDC is claiming attorney-client privilege.

DR. THOMPSON: No, they're trying to box you out.

DR. HOOKER: Yeah, that's fine . . . Sitting on a mountain, that's alright.

DR. THOMPSON: Here's what you have to do, honestly . . . and I'm telling you from the way I've changed my life. Here's what you have to do. You just have to try not to get emotions involved. Stay as settled and sound as you can be. Talk to people about how to market this fact that thimerosal causes tics. It's a marketing thing. It is all about marketing. And you have to learn, how do you get a message out? And I'm telling you, if you take autism out of it, you will get that message out. And once you get that message out, do you think a pregnant mother would take a vaccine that they knew caused tics?

DR. HOOKER: Absolutely not!

DR. THOMPSON: Absolutely not! I would never give my wife a vaccine that I thought caused tics.

DR. HOOKER: Right, right. That's genius. I mean, that's genius. You know, you've told me this before. It just didn't sink in.

DR. THOMPSON: But it's a marketing thing. It is a marketing thing. You have to figure out how to market this. And it has to come from other voices, it can't just come from you because you. . . They made you the poster boy of, they want to portray you as crazy and you know um and honestly, I think, you've been persistent. You have been right, I will say, most of the time. I will say the Geiers were not right and the Geiers . . . You know the Geiers; I do not know them personally. But, I know things they did. They took exact copies of papers we wrote and they published them under their own names. Word-for-word and I just thought that [UI].

DR. HOOKER: Yeah, I know a little bit about that but . . .

DR. THOMPSON: No, I just wanted to get back to that. Stay on message. Stay on a message that the press won't jump on. And get other people to say it. You have to get other scientists to say it because again, you're the poster child for this crazy person bothering the CDC making their life so difficult.

DR. HOOKER: Okay, okay. Hey, this has been extremely helpful. If you do get a chance, look at your SAS outputs and see if you ever did African American males.

DR. THOMPSON: Yeah, I'll forward you lots of programs.

DR. HOOKER: Awesome! Alright, thanks Bill. Good talking, bye bye.

DR. THOMPSON: Bye.

Chapter 3
Call 2

Second call: May 24, 2014
Thompson: "There is biologic plausibility right now,
I really do believe there is, to say that thimerosal causes
autism-like symptoms."

Sixteen days later, on May 24, Dr. Hooker called Dr. Thompson again to follow up on the original call.

* * * * * * * *

DR. HOOKER: Sorry about that. The best way for me to get return phone calls is if I use the restroom. I know that if use the bathroom a call will come, so. . . .

DR. HOOKER: How are you doin', man?

DR. THOMPSON: [*laughing*] I'm doing better, this has all been very stressful and uh, I finally got a lawyer, uh, on Monday. So, I'm (sic) at least have legal representative if anything blows up and uh, so that's good.

DR. HOOKER: Good, good, so that went well?

DR. THOMPSON: Yeah . . . My wife is not thrilled; she doesn't know anything about you and me. But she knows that uh ya know that the

Congressional stuff is getting very hot. And watching, she watched the Congressional hearings Tuesday morning and I watched them and uh . . . Posse [Posey] [*laughing*] is uh he seems like he is on the war path, so . . .

DR. HOOKER: He was not happy with Insel, that's for very sure, so um . . .

DR. THOMPSON: Yeah, and I didn't know about this study that Tom Insel was talking about and I asked Marshalyn [Yeargin-Allsopp] about it. She says she is going to find out for me. But I am going to find out. Do you know anything about this study?

DR. HOOKER: I have no idea what he was talking about. I heard that and ya know my initial thought was, "Well, the way he is talking about it I can predict what the outcome is going to be," but, going back to what you said previously, I'm sure they didn't look at tics.

DR. THOMPSON: Well let me tell you something really interesting I learned about this week so in the midst of this. Ya know, I was yelling at Marshalyn this week, I mean, Marshalyn and I were . . . WHOOOO! I was I suggested I resign and um is like that type of stuff going on right now. The whole place is a big pressure cooker . . . So I don't know if you know this. The CDC was invited to testify and they declined, so this is . . .

DR. HOOKER: Really?

DR. THOMPSON: Yeah, and Marshalyn said she's been offered to testify and said she won't. Coleen [Boyle] said she's been offered to testify and Coleen said that she would never go and testify again.

DR. HOOKER: And they don't subpoena. I mean, it's a very very rare instance that they would actually subpoena.

DR. THOMPSON: Really?

DR. HOOKER: Oh yeah. No, no, no, no. Rep. Issa doesn't like to use the subpoena unless he is really cornered to do so. It's just, it's one of the things that if he goes there too often then he comes under considerable criticism and he's trying to lobby for future chairmanship. Now he won't be the chairman. Most likely his term will be up in at the end of 2014. So 'cause it's a six-year term and he's had his six-years. But, no, they just don't like to do that. [Edited due to sensitive personal information.]

DR. THOMPSON: Right now I am sitting in a very pretty position in terms of providing you a lot of information and let me tell you what is um just became available and I was talking to Marshalyn and my team lead, my immediate supervisor, this week and I was telling them what should be done because it is just outrageous. You will die when you hear this.

We have eight hundred kids with autism that have been given the ADI, well that's autism diagnostic interviews for the parents, right, so, all of them have been give the ADI and the ADOS. So, they've all been given these instruments, all confirmed cases of autism. Um, we have population controls of similar size and we have disability controls of similar size. Now, this is the study I was brought in to clean up. Diana Schendel left town, left for Denmark, and I was brought in to clean it up. It's a big mess but regardless, there is now data available. Ya know, and there is going to be more data available. We're going to have twelve hundred kids with autism as part of this uh study, um, with all their medical records and all their vaccine records abstracted. So, um, what's amazing, now this is what's going to be shocking to you, it shocked the crap out of me. They have ya know six different sites interviewing data and um they all put in proposals to do studies. So far there is about sixty proposals in, um, for people ready to do studies. Not a single one of them looks at vaccines, not one! [*laughing*] So, I, well, I ripped into these people this week. And I'm like, "These vaccine studies have to be done. This is the largest case-control study you could ever do. They're all objectively identified as kids with autism. You have the vaccine records." And what I just, and I, after seeing the Posey hearing I was like, "What are you . . ." I was like, "How are you guys going to answer the question when you know they want these environmental studies and want to look at all these risk factors. What are you going to say when you have twelve hundred autism cases and a bunch of controls and you never looked at vaccines and you have all their vaccine records?" [*laughing*] . . .

DR. HOOKER: Oh my goodness . . .

DR. THOMPSON: And we have their prenatals, we have all the prenatal stuff that wasn't [unintelligible].

DR. HOOKER: I mean, this is like Disneyland.

DR. THOMPSON: It is like Disneyland. So here's the point, here's what I said to them. I said, I told them, "This study needs to be done." I said, "It should be contracted out to some independent organization," and I said uh, "Groups like SafeMinds should be included in the study and uh we [*laughing*] we're insane to be sitting on this data and not um ya know have an independent group, independent of the CDC, completely," I said. CDC not even touch it, not even have a coauthor on it. Anyway, so, the point I'm trying to make I want to give you the name of the study so you can start telling people who to ask questions about this study because this data is sitting ready to go. No one has analyzed it yet. And they don't really want people to know that this data exists, again. Ya know, you were the first person to get the MMR/autism—I just can't believe we actually got you that data.

DR. HOOKER: That's incredible to me. I'm very thankful; let's put it that way.

DR. THOMPSON: It's mind-boggling that um it sat on one CD and actually the guy that had the one CD just came down with pancreatic cancer. Literally, that study data could have been gone for good. Anyways, so the name of the study is The Study to Explore Early Development. It's called SEED. What?

DR. HOOKER: SEED? S-E-E-D.

DR. THOMPSON: Do you have a computer in front of you?

DR. HOOKER: Yes I do.

DR. THOMPSON: Just search for CDC and then SEED and then autism and you should be able to pull up a description of the study.

DR. HOOKER: Okay, hold on . . . SEED, autism spectrum disorders. Okay, there it is! Okay, let me bookmark this while I've got it.

DR. THOMPSON: Well that's the gold mine. That's the mother-load of mother-loads. Because it doesn't matter what Insel does. He doesn't have confirmed cases of autism in his study. His study will probably be some type of record review where they look at kids that have autism in the records.

DR. HOOKER: So, is this data that I would eventually be able to access myself?

DR. THOMPSON: Well, right now it's under lock and key and only the principle investigator can get to access it. But if you can get Posey to ask questions about this study, um, this will become, the, ya know, like [*laughing*] the leak in the dam.

DR. HOOKER: Oh my goodness, oh my goodness, here there is a tab on data and statistics that I am looking at okay and I see that, so. . . .

DR. THOMPSON: Now there's one study that has been published from it, just describing the study and the sample so, it is, Diana Schendel is the first author, 2012 paper, and you can just look it up. It might actually be on the website, I'm not sure. But, it's a Diana Schendel paper and it just pissed me off. I read it for the first time on Friday and she references two of her papers with Thorsen. I was just like, are you guys are fucking insane, I'm like, are you guys really this fucking insane.

DR. HOOKER: Well here it is. I looked it up on PubMed. It's in JADD, Journal of Autism and Developmental Disabilities.

DR. THOMPSON: That's the one paper that describes the first sample. There's SEED1 and SEED2.

DR. HOOKER: They piled it one. There's like twenty coauthors.

DR. THOMPSON: Yeah, it's all the PIs [Principal Investigators], everyone. It's a big study; there is six sites that are contributing data. But, it is the mother-load. Oh and then you know what else I found out this week? I almost went nuts.

DR. HOOKER: We can't have you do that again, dude!

DR. THOMPSON: No, I know. Do you know the name Lisa Croen?

DR. HOOKER: Yes I know Lisa Croen, she's in California.

DR. THOMPSON: She's with Northern California Kaiser. So, Diana Schendel is still involved in these studies. There are fifty proposals. One of the studies on um prenatal infection and I started asking questions. I'm like, "Who's doing the prenatal infections study?" She said, "Lisa and Lisa has invited Diana to participate." I'm like, "You are having Diana Schendel as a coauthor on a childhood infections paper while she's in Denmark with her boyfriend?!" [laughing] I just, you don't know how insane this all is. It's absolutely insane. Marshalyn and my supervisor is Laura Scheve. I don't know if you've seen that name.

DR. HOOKER: Yes, I've seen Laura's name before.

DR. THOMPSON: So anyways, the two of them are looking at them and they're like, "Maybe you're right; maybe that is a bad idea." [laughing]

DR. HOOKER: You think?! I think ya know Diana is putting herself in danger just by showing her head.

DR. THOMPSON: I could not believe that she was there. I could not believe she was there.

DR. HOOKER: Oh my goodness, that is just crazy.

DR. THOMPSON: So anyways, the bottom line is I want to get you the best data available. That is the best data available. No one has analyzed it yet. If you can get someone. And I just, Brian, you have to get someone other than you asking these questions because you are like, ya know, they just . . .

DR. HOOKER: I am damaged goods, I understand. No, and I do have some people in mind.

DR. THOMPSON: You just have to feed these questions around to different people and have different people ask these questions and ya know, so it's prenatal, I would tell there is both maternal influenza prenatal records; there's rhogam . . .

DR. HOOKER: Really, rhogam . . . okay.

DR. THOMPSON: Yeah, it's all there. Um, but I've never looked at it yet. But I could actually go into the database right now and do a frequency count on things. But, I'm not going to do anything like that right now. I'm just really trying to sort this all out. I'm trying to, ya know I'm being in trouble because I'm blowing up and stuff like that and I'm getting really agitated and I just have to settle down.

DR. HOOKER: Right, you had mentioned on I think on a previous voicemail something about maybe taking a leave of absence or um or uh putting in for a new assignment.

DR. THOMPSON: Yeah, I was considering getting detailed out of the branch. The downside to that is I would no longer have access to this type of information that I am sharing with you. I'm learning more and more. As I ask more and more, I'm learning more and more. I am, these people are like in one big bubble, they uh and their bubble is getting smaller and smaller. But, these PIs, it's two PIs that are really tight with Diana. That's Lisa Croen and Dani Fallin, you know, Dani Fallin F-A-L-L-I-N.

DR. HOOKER: That's a name that is not familiar to me.

DR. THOMPSON: She is a genetics expert and she is at Hopkins and um . . .

DR. HOOKER: And Lisa Croen as well.

DR. THOMPSON: Now Dani really likes Diana and is tight with Diana because we've been collecting genetic information from all of these subjects. All of these subjects have bloods drawn and swabs. Here's the other crazy thing, the CDC has not been able to get resources to sequence all these kids that we have. We have samples where you could sequence every single kid. And only a couple hundred have been sequenced and it is because Dani Fallin went and got money from the NIH. And I'm just like are you serious, you guys can't go out and get a small sum of money and it's not even a lot of money, it would just be like a couple of million dollars. And they could get every single kid sequenced; they're sitting on these. Yes, they're sitting on these samples.

DR. HOOKER: Can you imagine what we could do with them?

DR. THOMPSON: Oh my God! When I heard the Congressmen asking these questions, what are you guys doing? We are sitting on this gold mine. Here is the deal, the CDC is they're paralyzed. The whole system is paralyzed right now. And the whole branch is paralyzed and it's becoming more paralyzed. There's less and less and less being done as the place is coming to a grinding halt. Really, what we need is for Congress to come in and say give us the data and we're going to have an independent contractor do it and bring in the autism advocates and have them intimately involved in the study.

DR. HOOKER: Wow, I don't even know where to begin. I can definitely talk to Bill Posey about this.

DR. THOMPSON: Well, ask about this study; start asking questions about this study.

DR. HOOKER: I will, I will. And I will be able to sit down with him and explain what is going on with the study. And just ask questions. I don't want to appear to know too much. Just too much of a tip off. I wanted to take you back to something and if you don't want to talk about this, that's fine.

DR. THOMPSON: Let me just say one more thing. You saw that slide that I sent you?

DR. HOOKER: Yeah, the Barile presentation slides.

DR. THOMPSON: And you saw the last three slides, right? Did you see the reviewer's comments?

DR. HOOKER: [*laughing*] Did I ever?

DR. THOMPSON: No I know. And we were just trying to demonstrate that when this paper sat in clearance for over a year. The Birth Defects made us add the guy from Rochester as a coauthor. I've never been involved in a study like this before where I was asked to add a coauthor in the middle of clearance.

DR. HOOKER: So you were told that, get out! In the middle of the clearance process that then that guy was recruited?

DR. THOMPSON: Yes as the Birth Defects recommended that we add him as a coauthor um because they said we didn't know enough about tics so they added Ed Trevaithan's buddy, the guy at Rochester.

DR. HOOKER: So that's Ed Travaithan's friend?

DR. THOMPSON: Yep! So we added him and every step of the way, we had to water down the discussion and then we got it out and those reviewers, to give you an example of what happened, is that every single review said why are you not highlighting your significant [UI]. It was a unanimous opinion of the independent observers.

DR. HOOKER: I tell you, it made for good reading. It was pretty amazing and it seems like, without being too vicious, it seems like sort of a visceral response to a lot of people in CDC whenever they see a connection to an adverse event and a vaccine or a vaccine component.

DR. THOMPSON: No, I know. I actually presented it to Marshalyn's branch before I moved in there. I had Jack [Barile] present it and Jack and I prepared those slides and I was very happy that we put in that final slide that we confirmed ya know that thimerosal causes tics.

DR. HOOKER: You did and you've given me such a gift. I mean, that's such a hook in terms of getting thimerosal out of vaccines.

DR. THOMPSON: I am telling you, if people went around say that—do you think a mother?—And you and I have had this discussion already. And this is what blows my mind. What blows my mind is somehow, tics has not been added to the vaccine, ya know, the adverse events schedule.

DR. HOOKER: Right, it's definitely not a table injury.

DR. THOMPSON: But why?! Like, this is what I don't get. Like how, how there's, how are they? I started wondering like how does something get onto the table?

DR. HOOKER: And this is huge for me because my son has tics and he's in vaccine court.

DR. THOMPSON: I know, you told me. But how does something get onto the table? I don't get it.

DR. HOOKER: Oh, it has to go through HRSA. I don't know if it is ACCV that puts it on the table. But, it is very very difficult to get something on the table, I know that much.

DR. THOMPSON: Well anyway, you have that. You have that to support you now.

DR. HOOKER: Yes, I appreciate it. That was amazing. The other question I wanted to bring up was, two voicemails ago you talked about two individuals that I wasn't sure, if you don't want to answer this, that's fine. But, two individuals that you wanted to point out some of their activities or perhaps some of their behavior.

DR. THOMPSON: Well I [*laughing*], Brian, this is where you and I don't know each other very well and I . . . Here's what I struggle with, is I struggle with saying anything that isn't in writing that can't be backed up. Here's my fear okay? Let's say you go public with anything okay? Whatever and then it becomes clear that you got information from me. And then people will immediately say, "Well, he's mentally ill and why would you believe anything that he says, it's just hearsay."

DR. HOOKER: How do people know about your business? Why do they know about ya know . . . It's really none of their business your mental state or whether you're quote-unquote mentally ill or not.

DR. THOMPSON: I know but it will become, it will become, that will be the way they undermine me.

DR. HOOKER: I don't want that to happen, period.

DR. THOMPSON: No, I know but when I talked to this whistleblower lawyer, he said, "What do you want out of it?" and I said, "Well I just don't want to lose my job." And I said, "I'm willing to concede that I'll never do another autism study again if this all becomes public because obviously I can't be trusted to do that."

DR. HOOKER: Well, I would say in a perfect world that it would be the converse if this all became public. And I'm not saying anything that it will. That you would probably be the only person there that I would trust to do an autism study.

DR. THOMPSON: I know, maybe, maybe not, but I'm saying what he [Thompson's whistleblower lawyer] and I agreed to. This is a lawyer that was reading through these documents that had never seen them before. And I basically was telling this guy I was complicit, and I went along with this, we did not report significant findings. Ya know, I'm not proud of that and uh, it's probably, it's the lowest point in my career that I went along with that paper. [Edited due to sensitive personal information.]

DR. THOMPSON: When I talk to you [Dr. Hooker], you have a son with autism. I have great shame now when I meet families with kids with autism because I have been part of the problem.

DR. HOOKER: Not for my son personally. My son got his vaccinations in 1998, dude. You don't have to shoulder that one.

DR. THOMPSON: No, no, no, no. Here's what I shoulder. I shoulder that the CDC has put the research ten years behind. Because the CDC has not been transparent, we've missed ten years of research because the CDC is so paralyzed right now by anything related to autism. They're not doing what they should be doing because they're afraid to look for things that might be associated. So anyway there's still a lot of shame with that. So when I talk to a person like you who has to live this day in and day out, I say well, so I have to deal with a few months of hell if all this becomes public, um, no big deal. I'm not having to deal with a child who is suffering day in and day out. So that's the way I view all this. I am completely ashamed of what I did. So that's that.

DR. HOOKER: But you were told to do specific things.

DR. THOMPSON: Well, I, higher ups wanted to do certain things and I went along with it. I was in terms of chain of command, I was four out of five.

DR. HOOKER: Was it Melinda Wharton?

DR. THOMPSON: No, no, no, no. The coauthors.

DR. HOOKER: Oh, you mean Coleen [Boyle]?

DR. THOMPSON: Yeah, Coleen [Boyle] was the division chief, Marshalyn [Yeargin-Allsopp] was a branch chief, and Frank [Destefano] was a branch chief at the time. Now, Coleen is a center director, Frank is the director of immunization safety, and Marshalyn is a branch chief. They're still all much more senior than me. So, we're in a room discussing these things and there are things I haven't even shared with you because I can't prove it and that's what I struggle with. I don't want to share things with you that I can't prove that there aren't hard records because I am worried that the other four people will collude and say, "No, that's not true." So that's my fear.

DR. HOOKER: And it's your word against theirs and they're higher up . . .

DR. THOMPSON: Exactly. Well, they're higher up, four to one and I'm mentally ill. That's the picture that will be painted. Does that make sense?

DR. HOOKER: I wish it didn't.

DR. THOMPSON: But that's the way it will play out. That's why I'm trying to give you as many hard records as possible. And I think I've shared those last two that I sent to you. I don't know if you'd looked at them. Did you look at those results?

DR. HOOKER: Yes, I did.

DR. THOMPSON: You see that the strongest association is with those without mental retardation. The non-isolated, the non-mentally retarded, the effect is where you would think that it would happen. It is with the kids without other conditions, without the comorbid conditions. And the, ya know, honestly, I looked at those results, I had not gone through these hard copy papers, I don't think I have ever gone through them since 2004 and I came across them, and I'm like "Oh my God" and this is 0.97 to 16 and it's not statistically significant but odds ratio is 8 and if we would have added one more subject it probably would have been significant. I'm just looking that and I'm like. "Oh my God. I cannot believe we did what we did." But we did. It's all there. It's all there. I have handwritten notes.

DR. HOOKER: I understand your reluctance to name specific names because if you can't prove, it's your word against theirs.

DR. THOMPSON: It will be four to one and I will be the mentally ill guy.

DR. HOOKER: Yeah, it's criminal that well, it's criminal that they did a lot of things. But, it's criminal that they would, that what they do is if somebody falls out of line then it becomes personal, a personnel record and a personal issue.

DR. THOMPSON: Exactly, well, you saw the personnel record thing and I'm waiting for another personnel thing I mean ya know you wouldn't believe the things I've been doing this last week, this has all stressed me out a lot. My child has said to me today ya know, she's describing how crazy I've been over the last two weeks. But I am settling down. The good news is I am settling down.

DR. HOOKER: I need you sane.

DR. THOMPSON: I'm trying to stay sane. So what I'm trying to say is if you can put some of this off. Here's what scared the shit out of me, okay? When you said, have you sought legal counsel? When you said that, I'm like, oh no! Brian's going to go public really soon. So, it freaked the shit out of me. And that's why I got the lawyer.

DR. HOOKER: No, and quite frankly I have too much on my dance card to go forward with anything really soon. And so, no and I will give you the heads up before I do something like that.

DR. THOMPSON: Well I freaked and that's why I got a really good lawyer. So, I have a really good lawyer, in fact, he is going to do it pro bono. So, he is sitting, waiting and he's said when shit hits the fan, well give me a call and we'll seek everything out. So he has everything he needs. So I'm feeling that I am in a good spot but I need to settle down and what I want to tell you is if you could get people starting to ask questions. I'm sitting in a dream spot to basically give you feedback on how that information is playing out.

DR. HOOKER: That would be tremendous.

DR. THOMPSON: But there is this dream data set, I'm saying, this dream data set. But again, Brian, I don't know if vaccines cause a certain percentage or whatever. I can say [UI], I do think that thimerosal causes tics. I can say, tics are four times more prevalent in autism. There is a biological, there is biologic plausibility right now I really do believe there is, to say that thimerosal causes autism-like symptoms. And that's the way I say that.

DR. HOOKER: That's good enough.

DR. THOMPSON: And this whistleblower lawyer, the key thing he told me there's new whistleblower protections that went into effect November 2013. So in November, they added new language that protects scientists from giving their scientific opinion, they're allowed to give their scientific opinion and cannot be um ya know can't be punished.

DR. HOOKER: They can't be retaliated against. Okay, [UI] I did not know about that.

DR. THOMPSON: Oh my God, I was like oh my God. It went in right as I started sharing stuff with you [*laughing*].

DR. HOOKER: Wow, well that was the, that was first contact, was November 2013. So, then you have those rights.

DR. THOMPSON: So anyway. So I want to be a resource. I want to be valuable to you. I want you to have someone in the system that can give you feedback as these things go through and as long as you're willing uh ya know to let me to sit where I am I'll sit as long as I can tolerate it. And we'll just keep going.

DR. HOOKER: Okay, okay, well I appreciate it. You've given me a lot to think about. And let me really kinda explore this SEED website and then um, uh . . .

DR. THOMPSON: And get the paper, get the Diana Schendel paper.

DR. HOOKER: I will. I will. I've got access to JADD so I can do that.

DR. THOMPSON: Okay, great.

DR. HOOKER: Alright, thanks a lot, Bill.

DR. THOMPSON: Alright, good talking to you.

DR. HOOKER: Good talking to you, bye.

Chapter 4
Call 3

Third call: June 12, 2014
Thompson: ". . . these senior people [at CDC] just do completely unethical, vile things and no one holds them accountable."

Almost three weeks after the second recorded call, Dr. Hooker again called Dr. Thompson. Dr. Hooker now knows Dr. Thompson has hired a whistleblower attorney.

* * * * * * * * * * * * * * * * * *

DR. HOOKER: Are you there?

DR. THOMPSON: Yeah.

DR. HOOKER: Okay. I'm sorry. I'm about as bad as it gets on these phones, so . . . Um.

DR. THOMPSON: No problem.

DR. HOOKER: Trying to juggle two calls, it's like way beyond me. I always want to do the free conference call line, because that's a little easier, but ah . . . But so you're getting ready to head out for vacation?

DR. THOMPSON: Yeah, we're leaving tomorrow.

DR. HOOKER: Okay. Okay. Well, do you have time to talk tonight? I mean, I don't want to keep you too long, because you've got work in the morning.

DR. THOMPSON: Yeah, now is better than any other time, so why don't we talk now.

DR. HOOKER: Okay. Okay. I appreciate it. I wanted to talk to you about the MMR Study. I . . . Just to let you know, I wrote a paper on my results on MMR.

DR. THOMPSON: Yep.

DR. HOOKER: And that paper is out for peer review right now.

DR. THOMPSON: Yep.

DR. HOOKER: And what . . . I was thinking about this and it hadn't dawned on me before, but it will most likely include, you know depending on the peer review and everything, include something that I got from you. And I wanted to let you know that as soon as possible. I haven't heard back from the peer review; I'm not sure how long it's going to take. They have a web system. But one of the things that I demonstrated in the paper was that by taking the cohort of African Americans and then limiting it to only those that had the valid Georgia birth certificate that the relationship went away.

DR. THOMPSON: Yep.

DR. HOOKER: So, so, anyhow, I'll keep you apprised on that, but I'm concerned. I wanted to ask you a few questions. You had said earlier that . . . You were referring to the MMR Study, and you said something about being locked into specific analyses. And I wasn't sure what you meant. I thought, well, maybe you have an IRB, and they lock you in, you know, to what you're going to run . . .

DR. THOMPSON: Right, so let me just give you the three . . . There were the three studies. There was the . . .

DR. HOOKER: Sorry about the background, I don't know if you hear that; I'm up in a hotel at a Superfund Site for my other research, and this has been a crazy experience so far so.

DR. THOMPSON: Okay, but there were three big studies I worked on, okay?

DR. HOOKER: Okay.

DR. THOMPSON: There was the 2007 New England Journal paper, right?

DR. HOOKER: [Affirmative response.]

DR. THOMPSON: And we had an external panel of consultants that included Sallie Bernard.

DR. HOOKER: Right.

DR. THOMPSON: Then had the 2010 Price Autism Thimerosal paper, right?

DR. HOOKER: Right.

DR. THOMPSON: And we had an external panel that included Sallie Bernard.

DR. HOOKER: Right.

DR. THOMPSON: And let me just say for those two, for those two we agreed with the panel upfront what the analyses would be.

DR. HOOKER: Right.

DR. THOMPSON: And then we didn't deviate from those analyses. We presented them as we found them, and then we said, "We're making public use datasets, and people can go do additional analyses if they want."

DR. HOOKER: And you've done that.

DR. THOMPSON: Yeah, and we did that. Now with the MMR autism one, the . . . We had an analysis plan that we were supposed to execute, and it was written and, you know, I'm going to be sharing these draft analysis plans that we had and you can see whether we did what we said we're going to do.

DR. HOOKER: Right. What I'm trying to establish is if anything . . .

DR. THOMPSON: Let me just . . . Please just so you understand this, we didn't have an external review panel . . .

DR. HOOKER: Right.

DR. THOMPSON: . . . for the MMR autism one, so it was the one study where we could end up just replicating exactly what Tom Verstraeten ended up doing, which was just creating a mess while the CDC tried to, you know, tried to sort out something they couldn't understand.

DR. HOOKER: Right.

DR. THOMPSON: Right. Okay, so go ahead.

DR. HOOKER: Okay. You know, I want to . . . I'm thinking about this like a trial lawyer.

DR. THOMPSON: Yep.

DR. HOOKER: And, okay, down the road . . .

DR. THOMPSON: Yep.

DR. HOOKER: . . . this becomes public . . .

DR. THOMPSON: Yep.

DR. HOOKER: . . . and CDC says, "Well that's Bill Thompson; he's crazy."

DR. THOMPSON: Yeah, they will.

DR. HOOKER: And . . . But then we have a case that shows, okay, these are the analyses that you agreed upon and then you had your Verstraeten "Oh shit!" moment.

DR. THOMPSON: Yep.

DR. HOOKER: And then you basically deviated from that particular plan in order to reduce the statistical significance that you saw in the African American cohort.

DR. THOMPSON: Well, we, um, we didn't report findings that, um . . . All I will say is we didn't report those findings. I can tell you what the other coauthors will say.

DR. HOOKER: [Affirmative response.]

DR. THOMPSON: They'll say that the race variable was reliable is what they're going to say.

DR. HOOKER: But okay. Okay, playing that out, I mean as a statistician, that doesn't make any sense.

DR. THOMPSON: Well, I'm not going to defend it. I'm just trying to say . . .

DR. HOOKER: No, well I understand. I just think that if other coauthors were coming forward, were trying to dispute and say, "Well, we didn't think that that was a good . . . You know that the race was reliable." Then, you know, I'm trying to play that out, too, because when they say something like that they basically paint themselves in a corner.

DR. THOMPSON: Well, all I'm going to say is that they're going to say that.

DR. HOOKER H: Okay.

DR. THOMPSON: I know that is what they will say.

DR. HOOKER: Sure.

DR. THOMPSON: And I will tell you the only two people that can really answer that question will be Marshalyn or Coleen. Frank would not know that. I don't.

DR. HOOKER: [Affirmative response.]

DR. THOMPSON: I wouldn't know that, because I don't know that surveillance system.

DR. HOOKER: Right.

DR. THOMPSON: Tanja has left.

DR. HOOKER: Right.

DR. THOMPSON: And Tanja is gone. So the only two people who could defend that particular question would be Marshalyn or Coleen.

DR. HOOKER: Okay.

DR. THOMPSON: And that's all I can say.

DR. HOOKER: Okay, okay. Well, yeah, that makes sense. Okay. Okay. Now, on the runs you supplied the SAS programs . . . You supplied a lot of different SAS programs to me.

DR. THOMPSON: Yep.

DR. HOOKER: And I haven't tried to see if they'll run on SAS Enterprise Edition; I need to try that. But I was wondering, did you save any of your SAS output?

DR. THOMPSON: Yeah, I have SAS output but I only kept SAS output for the near final programs after we had, you know, gone through six to nine months of this—sorting through the results. So the only documentation I have are those Excel spreadsheets that were fed all these findings every time.

DR. HOOKER: Okay. Okay, but you don't have like the SAS listing file or . . .?

DR. THOMPSON: [Negative response.]

DR. HOOKER: Okay. Okay. I understand, so you've got . . . What was in the output is in the spreadsheets?

DR. THOMPSON: Every, every time we met, which was . . . You know, every time we met, I would create a new Excel spreadsheet, and I put in the new results in that Excel spreadsheet.

DR. HOOKER: [Affirmative response.]

DR. THOMPSON: And then we would meet and we would discuss them.

DR. HOOKER: Right.

DR. THOMPSON: Then I would go back and run more analysis.

DR. HOOKER: Right, right. Now going back to when the DeStefano Study was first initiated, what was . . . Was race a big factor? Because essentially what it appears in the final publication is that race in general is downplayed.

DR. THOMPSON: Of course it is.

DR. HOOKER: Right. It's downplayed. But was that a major objective in . . . And, you know, if you can show me what was planned in terms of the SAS runs, that's going to answer that question. But when you had the discussion . . . You know, I think of Metropolitan Atlanta, and I think, "Okay. This is a great place to get African Americans, because there's more African Americans that live in Atlanta than live in like Redding, California."

DR. THOMPSON: Yeah. Right. It would be the perfect city to do it, but as you can tell from the sample—and I think this is, in general, true at the time and it's still true—is that whites get diagnosed from that system that still exists and that we still publish, you know, the prevalence rates from—whites get diagnosed with autism at two times the rate of blacks.

DR. HOOKER: [Affirmative response.]

DR. THOMPSON: So, in 1996 when that was done, you know, that's before the big explosion.

DR. HOOKER: Right.

DR. THOMPSON: So, ah . . .

DR. HOOKER: I mean whites are getting diagnosed twice as much as blacks.

DR. THOMPSON: [Unintelligible.]

DR. HOOKER: There's not enough data really to do like a socioeconomic breakdown on that.

DR. THOMPSON: Well you can . . . I mean you can . . . You can . . . Well, did we include . . .? No. I don't think . . .

DR. HOOKER: No, no. There's any . . . I think there's like maternal education might be there.

DR. THOMPSON: Well, [UI]. This is the reason, is they were getting the records from the schools and from the clinics.

DR. HOOKER: Right.

DR. THOMPSON: So you don't have the sociodemographic data in there.

DR. HOOKER: Okay. Okay.

DR. THOMPSON: So, [UI], that brings up another interesting point, which I never even thought of. That's amazing, because, you know, the thimerosal studies, it was so important to get education and income, because there's a reverse association if you don't adjust for it.

DR. HOOKER: [Affirmative response.]

DR. THOMPSON: So . . . In fact, you could argue, you could argue the DeStefano paper is like a bunch of crap, because the better-educated moms get their kids vaccinated earlier. So, if we didn't adjust for that variable, you could argue from the other two studies, we had a crap study, because we weren't even adjusting for the appropriate variables.

DR. HOOKER: Right, right.

DR. THOMPSON: I never even thought of that.

DR. HOOKER: How would that play out? How would that play out? If better-educated moms then . . . If we do that, then basically what we're saying is, probably the level of education in the African American community for moms is going to be lower and so, therefore, they're probably going to get vaccinated later.

Dr. Thompson: Right. And, in fact, what this was suggesting is that among the blacks, the ones that were getting vaccinated earlier were more likely to have autism. Now the way that would play out if you thought of this bias, you would say, "The ones getting vaccinated earlier are the ones from higher-income backgrounds and, therefore, they could get . . ." I mean, if you just wanted to assume that bias was real . . .

Dr. Hooker: [Affirmative response.]

Dr. Thompson: . . . then you could argue that it's the educated black moms that are getting their kids vaccinated earlier and that's why you found that effect.

Dr. Hooker: And they're getting that effect and the ones that are getting vaccinated later are underdiagnosed.

Dr. Thompson: Yes.

Dr. Hooker: Okay. And not . . . And remembering that this was . . .

Dr. Thompson: But this is 1996 so . . .

Dr. Hooker: 1996 so the level . . . You know you didn't get early diagnoses then . . . The age cutoff was like between six and thirteen years of age, so I felt pretty comfortable using the whole cohort. I didn't feel like, "Oh, I need to exclude anybody because, you know, the average age of autism diagnosis . . ." But still . . . Yeah, that . . . I can see that, you know, that being a point that could be argued.

Dr. Thompson: Yeah.

Dr. Hooker: Okay. Okay. Good. Good to know.

Dr. Thompson: I didn't even think of it; I didn't even think of that until just now.

DR. HOOKER: Right. Right. Well, it does . . . You know, it does kind of play backwards . . .

DR. THOMPSON: Yeah.

DR. HOOKER: . . . in terms of: Will those kids that got vaccinated later; then you would expect less healthcare-seeking behavior; so they would be less likely overall to get an autism diagnosis.

DR. THOMPSON: Yep.

DR. HOOKER: But if you had the maternal education, then you could correct for that.

DR. THOMPSON: Right. But . . .

DR. HOOKER: So, I don't think I have it.

DR. THOMPSON: You could argue the most important confounder was not included in that study. So, why would you even consider the results valid?

DR. HOOKER: Valid. Right. Right, you can't say either way.

DR. THOMPSON: Exactly.

DR. HOOKER: Essentially.

DR. THOMPSON: Yep.

DR. HOOKER: You can't . . .

DR. THOMPSON: And you can use the other two studies to make that argument.

DR. HOOKER: [Affirmative response.] Well . . . But it's interesting, you know, because we don't see an effect whatsoever in whites. I mean, you take African Americans out of the mix so you don't see the effect in non-blacks period.

DR. THOMPSON: Yeah. I actually think the most interesting results are the elevated ones or the isolated—ones that don't have other comorbid conditions.

DR. HOOKER: Right.

DR. THOMPSON: So, what I think is interesting, because I've always believed that you would most likely find . . . If you could find an effect, you would find it among the ones without mental retardation . . .

DR. HOOKER: [Affirmative response.]

DR. THOMPSON: . . . because those are the ones where the results would be more sensitive. The kids without other comorbid conditions would be more likely to have something due to some exposure versus something that's just biological.

DR. HOOKER: Right. Right. So, biological . . . Something biological, then you would expect comorbidities . . .

DR. THOMPSON: Well, if you . . . The kids with mental retardation. . . .

DR. HOOKER: Right.

DR. THOMPSON: . . . it's probably, it's probably unlikely that mercury exposure causes mental retardation.

DR. HOOKER: How well though . . . If you've got . . . You know, and you, like you said before, you're not really the person to answer this but, how well do you have those records? Because a lot of times if you have an isolated autism case, you're going to have mental retardation. I don't . . . You know, I don't know; I'm out in the community; I don't really know many autistic kids that aren't mentally retarded.

DR. THOMPSON: Oh, I don't know. I actually don't know that for sure, but my reading of our own papers, the recent papers, is there's a huge increase in the number of kids who don't have mental retardation. That number is going, proportionately is going up.

DR. HOOKER: Right.

DR. THOMPSON: So, I still . . . I still say . . .

DR. HOOKER: But that could be . . . Part of that could be a health-care-seeking behavior, because if it's in vogue to get an autism diagnosis . . . And I deal with this as a parent all the time. You know, some genius walks up and tries to have a conversation with my kid, and I'll look at the parent and say, "Oh, my son has autism. He's non-verbal; he doesn't speak." And they'll look at me and they'll say, "Yeah, my kid has autism too." And I'm just like, "What the fuck! Really?" We should be so lucky to have that kind of autism.

DR. THOMPSON: Yeah. Well, I didn't know what type of autism your son had, so I did . . . I would . . . So, you know, many forms of retardation have a strong biological basis based on some, you know, prenatal insults or genetic predispositions.

DR. HOOKER: Sure.

DR. THOMPSON: So, I would just assume, and I may be assuming wrong, that if you have mental retardation, it's less likely going to be due to an environmental exposure.

DR. HOOKER: Right.

DR. THOMPSON: That environmental exposures are going to cause more subtle effects.

DR. HOOKER: Right.

DR. THOMPSON: This is my assumption, but I'm not . . . Again, don't . . . I can't . . .

DR. HOOKER: No, no, I understand. You know, you're not familiar with where that, that particular dataset. I mean you use the data, but you didn't . . .

DR. THOMPSON: Let me give you an example. What makes sense to me is that you would see something similar to the mercury fish exposure.

DR. HOOKER: [Affirmative response.]

DR. THOMPSON: You would see a couple of points, a couple of points decline in IQ, but you wouldn't assume that it'd be a fifteen-point decline on average, which would put a lot of people into the mental retardation category.

DR. HOOKER: [Affirmative response.]

DR. THOMPSON: But, you know, three or four IQ points, I could see that and that's essentially what lead does. Lead, you know, decreases your IQ . . . Lead exposure decreases your IQ by like three or four points.

DR. HOOKER: Right. Okay. Okay. Yeah. Yeah. This is making sense. Now . . . I want to switch gears here really quick. Going to the SEED data.

DR. THOMPSON: Yeah.

DR. HOOKER: How . . . You know . . . From my conversation I had with you back at the end of May, you have access to seed data, right?

DR. THOMPSON: [UI].

DR. HOOKER: You actually cleaned it up after Diana Schendel left, and so you have access to that database.

DR. THOMPSON: I have direct access to that data.

DR. HOOKER: Data. Okay. So, if I got, you know, a scientist that I would assume is trusted . . . You know, my . . . It would never be me in my wildest dreams as much as I would love to get into the SEED database, I'm not even going to think about it. In fact, I did access, I did request access to the public use data sets people, and they referred me to the State of Georgia SEED site.

DR. THOMPSON: Okay.

DR. HOOKER: I looked at the response and laughed and I thought, "Okay. This is what . . . This is what I expected." But if I had another trusted scientist, somebody like Cathy DeSoto, you know, for example; she's . . . You know, there's others. Is there a way to get them on the SEED team? You know, I, I . . . You had said, "Yeah. I could talk to Posey about it, and I have to talk to one of Posey's staffers," but is that team preassembled or . . .?

DR. THOMPSON: Well, here's the deal, and I've been having a lot of discussions about this. And it seems like I've sparked a conversation which I'm very happy about. So, there's the project officer who just does all the contract stuff for the studies.

DR. HOOKER: Right.

DR. THOMPSON: And she came to my office today and she said, "I heard you told Marshalyn that you think someone outside should do the vaccine studies." So it sounds like Marshalyn is trying to move forward on that idea.

DR. HOOKER: Oh wow.

DR. THOMPSON: But, you know, I think what Marshalyn wants is one of the principal investigators from one of the sites to take the lead. But as I told her, I said, "You should include outside groups with, ah, you know, opposing viewpoints." I'm like, "The CDC should not be involved at all; bring in outside people; let them be involved." Anyway . . . So it's really . . . I'm having this debate as we speak . . .

DR. HOOKER: Okay.

DR. THOMPSON: . . . about whether this system is an open system or a closed system, because I keep saying is, "If it is a closed system then Diana Schendel shouldn't be allowed to be coauthor on papers anymore. If it's an open system, then anyone should be allowed to use the data."

DR. HOOKER: Right; right. Regardless of what they've published in the past in terms of . . . Well, I mean, regardless of their good peer-reviewed science that they've published in the past; I'm not suggesting that we get Joe Schmoe who is inflammatory and . . . But good scientists . . .

DR. THOMPSON: Yeah. But I can promise you if you apply political pressure, things can happen.

DR. HOOKER: Okay.

DR. THOMPSON: And I promise you it will happen if you make Posey aware of that this is the largest case-control study in the world right now with objectively identified autism cases and all the exposures including vaccines . . .

DR. HOOKER: Right.

DR. THOMPSON: . . . and prenatal vaccines.

DR. HOOKER: Right.

DR. THOMPSON: It's, it's sitting there for the taking.

DR. HOOKER: Okay. Disney. Disney for this question so . . .

DR. THOMPSON: It is Disney; it is Disney on steroids relative to [UI] assessment.

DR. HOOKER: Right. Right. Well, what would happen . . . Okay, so let me play this out . . . My paper gets published; my MMR paper gets published. They . . . I get heavily criticized, because I haven't corrected for socioeconomic factors or maternal education. Yeah. I'll take my hits, and then eventually it gets published. And then there's a piece of information that I receive from the CDC, but I don't source. Is that going to be a red flag?

DR. THOMPSON: Say it again. If you do what?

DR. HOOKER: There's a piece of information, I have a piece of information saying that the CDC got this result and the CDC got this result on November 7, 2001.

DR. THOMPSON: Right.

DR. HOOKER: And then what they did was they took the . . . and they looked only at birth certificates or those individuals with Georgia birth certificates and that obviated that particular result. Okay. And so I report that. Now . . .

DR. THOMPSON: So, I have one question for you. Why are you using that particular date?

DR. HOOKER: Because that's the earliest date. That's the earliest date that African American effect was seen.

DR. THOMPSON: For some reason I don't think it was seen that early, but if you have . . . If I sent you a document that has that date, then that's the date but . . .

DR. HOOKER: It's in there. It was November 7, 2001. Yeah, it's in there.

DR. THOMPSON: Alright. I didn't think, I didn't think, I didn't think I had documented it that early. I thought it was several months later, but that's fine.

DR. HOOKER: Okay.

DR. THOMPSON: So, just say . . . You know, if someone asks, just say, you got it from Posey's office.

DR. HOOKER: Well, yeah. Well, you turned it over to Posey's office right? I mean you turned it over to people who were going to turn it over to Posey's office.

[Over talking.]

DR. THOMPSON: Yeah, I know, but I have no idea what they gave to Posey. And as you have been seeing from the emails I've been seeing, you know, they're coming up with every reason not to provide anything.

DR. HOOKER: Right.

DR. THOMPSON: A recent email suggested to me that they provided nothing previously on this MMR autism study. So, you know, right now I'm copying all those documents that . . . Any document I send to you, I'm turning into PDFs, and they'll all going to be PDFs, and I'm going to provide them as a part of this request.

DR. HOOKER: [Affirmative response.]

DR. THOMPSON: And I'm going to make it very clear that these were provided, because I have indications that they may have not provided everything this time around. So . . .

Dr. Hooker: Right.

Dr. Thompson: I'm trying to do everything I can to get it out the door. So anyways, I would just . . . If you get asked, I would just say you got it from [UI].

Dr. Hooker: Okay.

[Over talking.]

Dr. Thompson: . . . because you went in and you . . .

Dr. Hooker: I just want to, you know, if . . . I want to make sure that you're protected in this and, you know, this is probably a crazy idea. But I was thinking if there would be a possibility that you could go on the record, like a private deposition with your whistleblower attorney, and you could say, "This and this and this and this. This is the sequence of events and, by the way, what they're going to say is that I'm a crazy person because of this, this, this and this." You know, do you remember Benazir Bhutto? She was the prime minister of Pakistan. She was killed. She was killed by terrorists.

Dr. Thompson: Yep.

Dr. Hooker: And about two months before her murder, she got up in public and said, "Oh, by the way, if I'm killed? It will be by these people and this is how they're going to do it and this is how they'll get away with it."

Dr. Thompson: Yeah.

Dr. Hooker: And so she basically went on record, and she anticipated based on what she knew what was going to happen, and then was able to out the people that killed her.

Dr. Thompson: Yeah.

Dr. Hooker: So, I'm just wondering if there's a way that coming down the pike, if you can anticipate some of the persecution, that the potential for persecution if there's a way for you to go on record to say, "This and this and this; this is the sequence of events of what happened and this could possibly happen to me."

DR. THOMPSON: I don't want to go down that road. [Edited due to sensitive personal information.]

DR. HOOKER: Right.

DR. THOMPSON: So here's what . . . At this point, I'm just trying to get comfortable with everything I've shared with you, I can share with you. I don't take a stand on anything, and you have what you have. You're going to do what you're going to do with it.

DR. HOOKER: Right.

DR. THOMPSON: And, you know, I've tried to share with you as much information as possible. And if you say you spoke to me, I promise you, everyone will paint me out to be the bad guy, and they'll dig up stuff. And I'll become the story about why I've become the next Brian Hooker and can't be listened to.

DR. HOOKER: Yeah, see, see . . . In thinking about history and posterity and all that type of stuff, I wouldn't . . . I can't foresee doing that to you.

DR. THOMPSON: No, no, no, no. I'm just saying . . . I'm just playing it out.

DR. HOOKER: Right.

DR. THOMPSON: Like if you play it out, I would just become the next Brian Hooker. I would be the next scapegoat for the drug companies.

DR. HOOKER: What about those, what about those inside that are sympathetic with you? I mean, do they exist?

DR. THOMPSON: I don't think there's anyone sympathetic inside to what I am doing or what I have . . . My position is one that the drug companies will jump all over. I mean . . .

DR. HOOKER: Sure.

DR. THOMPSON: I mean, they . . . Right now, they feel like they have you pretty isolated as an extremist and, so . . .

DR. HOOKER: Yeah, I know. I checked my Wikipedia entry the other day and I saw what kind of extremist I was. I actually had to like become a member of Wikipedia, so I could edit what was said about me.

DR. THOMPSON: I said you've got to do that too and it's gonna happen. But . . . Just so you know. So in the short term, I'm not going to leave the federal government. I . . . Again, I don't think, based on everything I know right now, I don't think I've broken a single law.

DR. HOOKER: No. No.

DR. THOMPSON: I'm . . . Nothing I shared with you is classified; nothing I shared with you is privileged information in any way. And if anything, people that have been my supervisors have broken laws. And . . . But I'm not going to be the judge of that. So . . .

DR. HOOKER: Why not? I'm sorry. That's . . . I meant to put you on the spot. If you feel on the spot, mission accomplished. But if they're doing things that are illegal that are hurting children, I mean . . .

DR. THOMPSON: I know, but I'm . . . I'm . . .

DR. HOOKER: But I understand the quandary if you can't prove it. If you can't prove it, you can't prove it. And you can't go on record, because they're going to make you look like shit.

DR. THOMPSON: No, again, it's gonna turn into hearsay. It's going to be my opinion versus four other coauthors.

DR. HOOKER: [Affirmative response.]

DR. THOMPSON: And the four [UI] coauthors have a lot of support from the rest of the CDC. There is no one that would come to my defensive. The rest of them are all senior-level people, and everyone would rally around them and try and figure a way out. And they would figure a way out. That's the deal. That's the, that's what I keep seeing again and again and again, and I've been involved in the separate situation unrelated to this, where these senior people just do completely unethical, vile things and no one holds them accountable.

DR. HOOKER: Does it have to do with vaccine safety? Or?

DR. THOMPSON: No, no, no, no; this is completely unrelated. Nothing to do with it.

DR. HOOKER: Unrelated? Okay, Okay. I'm not going to pursue it then. Um, then, um, because it's, it's not, this is not isolated to DeStefano, DeStefano et al. 2004. I mean I've got all the records. I see that on the New England Journal of Medicine paper, you were pressured to downplay the relationship between thimerosal and tics.

DR. THOMPSON: Well, I, I uh, let me just say this. I did a follow-up study, because I wanted my opinion on the record.

DR. HOOKER: Right.

DR. THOMPSON: I talked to a graduate student outside the CDC to analyze the data, so it wouldn't even be me who was leading it.

DR. HOOKER: Right.

DR. THOMPSON: And then I went through this process where that paper was in clearance for a year, and where I was asked to bring a coauthor on in the middle of clearance, which is one of the most . . .

DR. HOOKER: Right, right. The guy from Rochester. Yeah.

DR. THOMPSON: . . . [UI] things you can do. Yeah. So the point is . . . Well here's, here's where I think and, it's almost impossible to prove because I've already heard people respond to it, but, I've said things like, "Why didn't you guys follow up on the significant thimerosal effect?" And it went into the NVPO plan. They spent almost two years writing the plan on what they would follow up on. They were supposed to follow up on tics, and they never did a single additional study on tics. So, they were supposed to follow up on this. That was the one thing I wanted to see if they would follow up on and they never did.

DR. HOOKER: See the NVPO is like Fort Knox when it comes to FOIA.

DR. THOMPSON: No, I know. But the bigger problem is they're not actually following up on things they say they're going to follow up on.

DR. HOOKER: Right, right. See there was a concerted effort not to look at it. Because if they were going to follow up on it, then that would have been as part of the 2011 IOM . . .

DR. THOMPSON: Yeah.

DR. HOOKER: . . . and the 2013 IOM, and they didn't look at thimerosal whatsoever. They were just like, "Okay, you know what, if we don't talk about this, then the final word will be 2004." And you know, they said, "Thimerosal does not cause autism and that's the end of it."

DR. THOMPSON: I know. But like I said, they never say, "Thimerosal does not cause tics."

DR. HOOKER: Right, Right. Which we do have a plan for, by the way. I mean, you will see something out in the press hopefully by the end of this month.

DR. THOMPSON: Okay. Good. Because that should be your mantra. That should be your mantra.

DR. HOOKER: That is, that is, that is our mantra. It's been very, very, you know, difficult to get through but, yes, it is our mantra. The thing that, the medical community seems to think that on the developmental disability scale, that tics are bottom feeders. That's like, "Oh no big deal, no big deal."

DR. THOMPSON: The question is, "What is it linked to? What is it represented about?"

DR. HOOKER: Right.

DR. THOMPSON: It's the canary in the coal mine is what it is. It's a manifestation of an exposure that may have had a lot of other effects such as verbal learning problems, which were also found in several studies.

DR. HOOKER: Right, right. And that's . . . Yeah, I found a study that basically said that there were Learning Disability [LD] comorbidities in 76 percent of the cases of tics.

DR. THOMPSON: Right.

DR. HOOKER: So, there was ADHD, ADD, behavioral regulations, speech and language delay, and autism.

DR. THOMPSON: Which I'm very impressed you dug up that one tic and mercury exposure thing. I'd never seen that. That was . . .

DR. HOOKER: Yeah, it was methyl mercury in a Chinese herbal spray.

DR. THOMPSON: Yep. [UI].

DR. HOOKER: Yeah, yeah. It was very interesting. And then as the blood mercury levels dropped, then they saw the tics subside.

DR. THOMPSON: Right. I mean I think that's a wonderful demonstration. I was going to ask you this. So, for a couple interesting rat studies that I read a while ago, in one of the studies that was interesting was, they were trying to find the toxic level of thimerosal to see how they would do a study. And I've never seen anyone replicate it, but I thought it was a really interesting study and it could be replicated really easily. So, they took male and female rats and were trying to find out the toxic dose that would essentially kill them before they lowered the dose to see the effects of thimerosal. Well, in this one study that is in the literature, all the males died and the females didn't. So, they got to a certain level and all the male rats died. So to me . . .

DR. HOOKER: Wow.

DR. THOMPSON: . . . again, it showed that thimerosal had a differential effect on males and females, which would be consistent with, you know, whatever . . .

DR. HOOKER: With a lot of LD, not just autism. But with a lot of LD. So . . .

DR. THOMPSON: Yeah, yeah, yeah.

DR. HOOKER: Okay.

DR. THOMPSON: It was fascinating.

DR. HOOKER: Can you send me the reference for that?

DR. THOMPSON: I can try and dig it up. I'm sure I can find it again but . . .

DR. HOOKER: Okay. I appreciate it. So. But getting back to this. You had our favorite person, Tanja Popovic.

DR. THOMPSON: Yep. She may have resigned. No one will say whether she really resigned or not. Did she resign?

DR. HOOKER: I don't know. I'm supposed to get a [UI]. That was part of my Posey request was to get all of her emails that said thimerosal or autism.

DR. THOMPSON: Yeah.

DR. HOOKER: And I wanted to get it in there really quick, because I thought, you know, "I have a two-week window and all those emails will just be down the drain." If that.

DR. THOMPSON: Yeah.

DR. HOOKER: How does it work? Is it an issue when it goes through clearance? Or, that it gets bounced back? Or?

DR. THOMPSON: That what gets bounced back?

DR. HOOKER: That if they see an effect, that then they will bounce it back to you during the clearance process or you know if, for example, what you said for the Barile paper. That it was in clearance, and then they wanted you to get this second author or this additional author.

DR. THOMPSON: It was a very, very, very rare—I've never seen it happen before. So that's the first time I've ever seen something like that happen before. But they had no knowledge that this was coming through versus the two thimerosal studies. Those people knew about the results like, you know, two years before it went into clearance.

DR. HOOKER: [Affirmative response.]

DR. THOMPSON: So almost . . . Well, I would say every study that has ever come out on immunization safety, the people above know. . . . If there's a significant finding, they know months in advance of it going into clearance. So, my paper, I put into clearance without them knowing anything about it, and it caught people off guard, and then we went through the process we went through which was a slow, laborious. But I kept pounding away; they kept watering it down. They watered it down. Then we sent it out to the journals. And the journals were just like, "What the fuck?"

This watering down during clearance confused the reviewers at the journal. Why would the authors of a paper containing a significant finding want to water that finding down during clearance?

DR. HOOKER: [Affirmative response.]

DR. THOMPSON: You're not even talking about the significant finding you found.

DR. HOOKER: Right, right. The three reviewers said that the page on that Power Point presentation, that's dynamic. I mean, that's radioactive.

DR. THOMPSON: Yeah.

DR. HOOKER: And it's such an indictment.

DR. THOMPSON: Yeah. It's an indictment of the whole process.

DR. HOOKER: Right. Right.

DR. THOMPSON: Yeah.

DR. HOOKER: So did you feel in the 2007 paper that you were pressured to downplay significant results?

DR. THOMPSON: No. Because in both those cases, AFT had the results and they presented them . . . I mean myself and Sallie Bernard saw them, the results, for the first time at the same time.

DR. HOOKER: Put Sallie Bernard off the table; she's a double agent. You know that. She's no friend of the autism community. Period.

DR. THOMPSON: I have no idea but . . .

DR. HOOKER: No, she's not. She basically wants . . . She's this uber-rich lady that wants to talk about how she's helping autistic kids, so she can parade around the cocktail party circuit. If I see Sallie Bernard on one more CDC panel, I'm going to spit up and send it to you.

DR. THOMPSON: I see.

DR. HOOKER: I'm sorry. [Edited due to sensitive personal information.]

DR. THOMPSON: But she's a political animal. I mean. She . . .

DR. HOOKER: She is.

DR. THOMPSON: Right? So that's why she was on the panel. But she was sort of, the token representative of the anti-vaccine contingent.

DR. HOOKER: [Affirmative response.] Contingent, right, right.

DR. THOMPSON: So, she was supposed to represent that contingent and . . . So anyway, so when they presented the results to me, I was seeing them at the same time she was. I was, you know, we were all shitting in our pants. Those two studies . . .

DR. HOOKER: [Affirmative response.]

DR. THOMPSON: . . . we didn't know what we were going to see when we showed up into the room.

DR. HOOKER: Right.

DR. THOMPSON: So, I was very happy about that. I was happy that we wouldn't be able to spin it. That it was put on the table, and Sallie could walk away with a handout of the results. And she actually . . . I don't think she released the results to the public till after it was published by [UI].

DR. HOOKER: No, she didn't. She didn't. So, it . . . I was trying to get the results. I was trying. I wasn't getting them from her. I was trying to get them from the FOIA. But, no, those weren't released. And, you know, understandably so. I mean, in looking at the FOIA exemptions, I understand why and it wouldn't be defensible. You know, I couldn't go to court to get those results prior to publication. They would be considered pre-decisional.

DR. THOMPSON: Right.

DR. HOOKER: . . . So . . .

DR. THOMPSON: So anyway, so anyways . . . So, it did . . . You know . . . I don't know how we got on that topic.

DR. HOOKER: Oh, that's all alright. I'm sorry. That was me. I dragged you over there. Sorry.

DR. THOMPSON: So to answer your question, there was no pressure on those two studies because essentially, AFT handed us a book of results, and then we wrote up a paper based on that book. Right?

DR. HOOKER: [Affirmative response.]

DR. THOMPSON: We all show up in the room. Everyone gets handed a book. The book is the book. And then we write up the papers. It was like, the most straight-forward thing in the world because everyone agreed upfront what the analysis would be. A book comes in. It has everything, and then we write it up and publish it.

DR. HOOKER: [Affirmative response.]

DR. THOMPSON: It was very different from this other process where we spent, where we were just wondering I mean . . . And then when I find out what was going on in the background with these other studies with Diana Schendel, I'm like, "Oh, that's where . . ."

DR. HOOKER: Right.

DR. THOMPSON: We're wondering while she's money laundering with the person that's, you know, the landmark study that dismisses any association.

DR. HOOKER: Exactly; exactly.

DR. THOMPSON: I mean, she spent the summer in Denmark the year she published that study. You know . . .

DR. HOOKER: The . . . Which one are you referring to? I'm sorry. I should know this.

DR. THOMPSON: Her 2003 and 2004 papers.

DR. HOOKER: Oh Madson 2000 . . . She spent the summer for Madson 2003?

DR. THOMPSON: She spent the . . . She took a summer and essentially vacationed in Denmark. I'm sure she said she was working, but . . .

DR. HOOKER: I could tell you stories about that study. Oh my goodness.

DR. THOMPSON: Yeah.

DR. HOOKER: It is . . . You know, they cherry picked data. They . . . well, Madsen (2003) is . . . It's so fatally flawed.

Dr. Thompson: Yeah.

Dr. Hooker: You know with the changing diagnostic criteria; the inclusion criteria regarding clinics; the inpatient versus outpatient. I mean, it's such a mess.

Dr. Thompson: No, I know. But I'm just saying, while I'm out defending a dissertation on a weekly basis, she's out in Denmark money laundering with her boyfriend.

Dr. Hooker: Yes, party at Thorsen's house. Okay.

Dr. Thompson: Sitting at the seaside with Thorsen . . .

Dr. Hooker: Right.

Dr. Thompson: . . . and his Harley, and his second house in Atlanta.

Dr. Hooker: Did you? You know, going back to Thompson, did . . . Was maternal education and . . .? That was a covariant in that one, right?

Dr. Thompson: Yeah.

Dr. Hooker: And maternal age?

Dr. Thompson: Yep.

Dr. Hooker: Okay. Were those strong covariants? Do you remember?

Dr. Thompson: Yes. They were very strong.

Dr. Hooker: They were very strong. Okay. Okay, that makes sense. I'm just wondering though . . . The majority of the metrics though were tested, they were tested; you know by, interviewed by folks that were employed by [UI] associates.

Dr. Thompson: They were all brought in for a three-hour neuro psychologically test [UI]. A group of masters-level training folks were all . . .

Dr. Hooker: Okay.

DR. THOMPSON: . . . taught in a standardized way to give a full neuro-psych test battery.

DR. HOOKER: Okay.

DR. THOMPSON: They brought the kids . . . The kids were brought in for three hours at the three or the four different HMOs that participated, and the family was invited in. The kid would be given a three-hour test. You know, sat down and give them IQ tests and all that type of stuff.

DR. HOOKER: Sure.

DR. THOMPSON: And the mother was given a short, just quick IQ test that we use as the covariant, and I'm telling you, it was very labor intensive and that study was done really well.

DR. HOOKER: Right.

DR. THOMPSON: Yep.

DR. HOOKER: Right. It and Barile 2012 stand alone.

DR. THOMPSON: They were as good as you could do. I will say in hindsight, I think it was a big mistake to wait until they were seven years old to test them because again, mercury exposure, there's other things. You and I talked about this. There's other things that could come in. You know, people with financial resources could bring in things to essentially ameliorate any deficits that might have occurred.

DR. HOOKER: Right. Yeah, that makes sense. I mean, the socioeconomic status is going to work for . . . Well, healthcare-seeking behavior is a moot point because you're testing everybody. You're levelling the playing field. But, socioeconomic factors could weigh in otherwise in test scores.

DR. THOMPSON: Yeah. Between birth and seven years.

DR. HOOKER: Right.

DR. THOMPSON: So personally, if I was going to redo it, I would've done it at three years of age or four years of age.

DR. HOOKER: 'Cause it makes sense.

DR. THOMPSON: At that point, that would probably be the earliest point you'd start seeing deficits show up. And it would be before you'd get a lot of early intervention education stuff that people with resources could do.

DR. HOOKER: Sure, sure. It makes sense. So, you weren't involved in Verstraeten in 2003 at all, were you?

DR. THOMPSON: No.

DR. HOOKER: You laugh. Yes. Yes.

DR. THOMPSON: That was a circus; that was a total circus. And then he goes to the IOM . . .

DR. HOOKER: Right.

DR. THOMPSON: . . . [UI] to give this presentation that he's going to work for a drug company. I mean that was as dark as [former CDC Director] Julie Gerberding going to work for Merck vaccine. I mean, it was just . . .

DR. HOOKER: Right, right. That's, that's. . . .

DR. THOMPSON: Nothing pissed me more than him doing that.

DR. HOOKER: I'm sorry?

DR. THOMPSON: Nothing pissed me off more than him doing that at the IOM Meeting. Saying, "I now work for a drug manufacturer."

DR. HOOKER: Yeah. He basically resigned on stage.

DR. THOMPSON: And it was a total slap in the face. It's just like, how insulting would that be to these people who are looking for an unbiased viewpoint?

DR. HOOKER: Right. Well yeah. It had, it had a dramatic chilling effect. Let's put it that way.

DR. THOMPSON: Well. I wouldn't believe another word coming out of someone's mouth who, on stage says, "Oh, and today I accepted a job with a drug manufacturer."

DR. HOOKER: Yeah. No. No. He was done. As soon as he said that, he was done. You're right. You're absolutely right. But . . . So . . . Okay. You know, you and I are in agreement. Vaccine safety should not be in the CDC.

DR. THOMPSON: Absolutely.

DR. HOOKER: So how do you see this all ending? I mean, how would this end? How . . .

DR. THOMPSON: Right. It would end this way. That you would end up with an agency like the National Transportation Safety Board. You know, the FAA; then there'd be NTSB. The FAA is responsible for regulating all sorts of things, but then when an accident happens, you bring in the NTSB. So, you would have the equivalent of an NTSB-like organization that would do vaccine safety studies independently.

DR. HOOKER: Right.

DR. THOMPSON: And, um, but here's the . . .

DR. HOOKER: But how do we get there? I mean my fundamental question is, "How do we get there?" We are here now.

DR. THOMPSON: Right.

DR. HOOKER: How do we get there? I mean, without shrapnel, preferably.

DR. THOMPSON: You know, I'm becoming skeptical of these things as I look at it over time because I look at the Environmental Protection Agency . . .

Dr. HOOKER: Right.

Dr. THOMPSON: . . . and it seems like they're being watered down. They're being less and less effective. So I just think the trend right now is toward not allowing the government to say anything negative about any industry. So . . .

Dr. HOOKER: Right. So it's going on with the USDA with the Monsanto Protection Act. You know.

Dr. THOMPSON: Yeah.

Dr. HOOKER: Trust me. I genetically modify plants for a living. That's what I did. That's how I cut my teeth on my research, post, you know, essentially what would be referred to as my postdoc years at the National Laboratory was . . .

Dr. THOMPSON: [Affirmative response.]

Dr. HOOKER: You know, you don't want to eat GM food. You don't want to eat round-up ready anything. And because Monsanto is now the insider.

Dr. THOMPSON: Yeah.

Dr. HOOKER: You know, they're the government insiders and the environment is getting increasingly hostile for those that would speak out within the government that would speak out against the government.

Dr. THOMPSON: Yes. Exactly. So that seems to be the trend. So, I just don't think the time is right right now or you're not going to get a lot of—believe it or not, when Bob Chen was the Grants Chief at Immunization Safety, he was the one that was pushing really hard to get Immunization Safety moved out of the CDC. I think he actually almost succeeded, but then they reprimanded him and slapped him around and . . .

Dr. HOOKER: Transferred him.

DR. THOMPSON: Yeah. And then moved him out.

DR. HOOKER: Right. Right.

DR. THOMPSON: So I just think the current environment in the federal government and you know this because you were in the federal government . . .

DR. HOOKER: Right.

DR. THOMPSON: . . . is hostile to anyone who says anything negative about any industry. So I don't know what the answer is. I don't know how we get independent studies. What I want to say is, "The NIH should be funding all the studies," is what I want to say.

DR. HOOKER: [Affirmative response.]

DR. THOMPSON: But I'm beginning not to trust the NIH with vaccine studies you know.

DR. HOOKER: Sure. Sure. Some of the comments that Tom Insel made, you know, he had a preconceived notion of how his quote/unquote "Vaccine Safety Study" that he was working on, his VAC/UNVAC study was going to come out. I mean, to be very, very clear . . .

DR. THOMPSON: Have you heard any more about that? Have you asked anyone about that study?

DR. HOOKER: I haven't heard anything. Not for lack of time, I haven't heard anything about that study. I may . . . call Lyn Redwood . . . because she's on IACC and she might know.

DR. THOMPSON: Yeah.

DR. HOOKER: So, I may call her.

DR. THOMPSON: I mean, I asked Marshalyn and Marshalyn didn't know.

DR. HOOKER: No. No. I'm not sure who is doing what. But if it's anything like that one meta-analysis that came in Australia, good luck. You know.

DR. THOMPSON: Oh God. That meta-analysis was the saddest paper I've ever seen. The amount of press that piece of crap paper got was so depressing.

DR. HOOKER: Right.

DR. THOMPSON: It just . . . It was mind-numbing to think how much press that got which described it as a nail in the coffin. [Frustrated noise.] Anyway. [Edited due to sensitive personal information.]

DR. HOOKER: Okay. Okay. That's it man. It's late.

DR. THOMPSON: Have a good night.

DR. HOOKER: Alrighty. Hey, thanks a bunch WB. We'll talk to you soon.

DR. THOMPSON: [UI].

DR. HOOKER: Bye-bye. Have a great vacation.

Chapter 5
Call 4

4th call: July 28, 2014

Thompson: "I'm telling you. I did [send] a hundred
thousand pages [to Congressman Posey's office]."

The fourth and final recorded call is almost seven weeks after
the third call. During the second call, Dr. Hooker learned that
Dr. Thompson hired a whistleblower attorney. During the third
call, Dr. Thompson learned that Dr. Hooker was on the verge of
publishing a paper about the 2004 MMR study.

✱ ✱ ✱ ✱ ✱ ✱ ✱ ✱ ✱ ✱ ✱ ✱

DR. HOOKER: Hello.

DR. THOMPSON: Hey Brian.

DR. HOOKER: Hey, how you doing?

DR. THOMPSON: Alright. How are you?

DR. HOOKER: Good. Just trying to figure out how to use the new
iPhone 5 that I got; my plan finally upgraded. It took me two frickin
years, but I finally upgraded to a normal phone. Yeah, how's your
summer going?

DR. THOMPSON: Oh, it's going pretty good. We were in Chicago last week for vacation; that was good.

DR. HOOKER: Oh wow. You've got family there, right? You're pretty close to Wisconsin and Chicago.

DR. THOMPSON: Yeah. A brother and sister that live in Chicago and the kids were in a Blues camp and . . .

DR. HOOKER: A Blues camp, that's awesome.

DR. THOMPSON: Yeah. It was really fun and they got to play in The House of Blues which was really cool.

DR. HOOKER: What do they play? They're both instrumental musicians?

DR. THOMPSON: Yeah. My son plays the drums. My daughter plays electric guitar and lead singer.

DR. HOOKER: Oh, no way.

DR. THOMPSON: Yeah.

DR. HOOKER: Now I know what your retirement plan is. They just need to get famous.

DR. THOMPSON: Well, we joke about the lake house. They're going to get it.

DR. HOOKER: That's good. Well, well . . . My son and I . . .

DR. THOMPSON: Well, how are you doing?

DR. HOOKER: Good. . . . we hit a deer.

DR. THOMPSON: Yeah.

DR. HOOKER: I don't know if I told you that.

DR. THOMPSON: No.

DR. HOOKER: We were up in the mountains. Up north of Redding, toward Mount Shasta. And my son is really into instrumental music, only like marching bands.

DR. THOMPSON: [Affirmative response.]

DR. HOOKER: And so there are these professional marching bands called Drum and Bugle Corps, and there was one practicing up . . . They practice up in the mountains, because it's the only place in California that actually gets cool. And so, we were up there checking them out practicing, and we headed home. We had like a sixty-mile drive home and pasted a deer right at dusk. In fact, I never saw it.

DR. THOMPSON: How fast were you going?

DR. HOOKER: About sixty-five. It was on the freeway.

DR. THOMPSON: Oh my gosh.

DR. HOOKER: It was horrible. [UI].

DR. THOMPSON: So what happened?

DR. HOOKER: Well we had a '96 Ford Explorer that's what we hit it in. And those things are pretty impervious, so we were okay. But the airbags deployed and that alone was wild.

DR. THOMPSON: Oh.

DR. HOOKER: I never . . .

DR. THOMPSON: Did you airbag burn that everyone talked about?

DR. HOOKER: Yep. Yep. You're the first person that's actually nailed it. No, we had burn marks. We had bruises. And the stuff, the stuff that they use to get it to inflate just stinks to high heaven.

DR. THOMPSON: Yeah, I've heard that. Yeah.

DR. HOOKER: It smells like diesel and skunk. It is just awful.

WT: Aww. How'd your son react to it?

DR. HOOKER: He did really well, and I was so thankful because I don't know what we would've done if . . . You know, if I would've passed out, he would've wandered off because we were in the woods.

DR. THOMPSON: Oh, oh . . .

DR. HOOKER: And, so, you know, I was lucid; I checked on him; he was fine. We got out of the car because the horn was stuck on and because of his sound sensitivity and just because of the stink; it just smelled so bad in the car. But then once we got to the side of the road, we actually . . . I never saw the deer until after we hit it. So we're on Interstate 5 and all these big semis keep on re-hitting the deer that we killed and this deer shrapnel is flying up and hitting us. But we finally . . . It took us . . . The tow truck, the squad car came, and my son got to sit in the back of the squad car and he liked that. He dug that. And then the tow truck came and actually took us the wrong direction so we had to spend the night in the mountains, and my wife came and got us the next day.

DR. THOMPSON: Oh . . .

DR. HOOKER: So, it was good. It was a fun experience.

DR. THOMPSON: When did that happen?

DR. HOOKER: Oh, that was probably the end of June—around that timeframe. And . . . But I got a new Ford Explorer; I'm not complaining. I got one with less miles, so you know, I'm . . .

DR. THOMPSON: Covered by insurance, covered by insurance or what?

DR. HOOKER: Exactly; exactly. So, we had to put in about two thousand of our own bucks, but, yeah, that was fine. It worked out okay. But, anyhow, I'll tell you what, the reason why I wanted to talk to you is that I have been in Issa's office . . .

DR. THOMPSON: Yep.

DR. HOOKER: . . . and I've seen your handy work.

DR. THOMPSON: Which part of it? Which part of it? Okay. Go ahead.

DR. HOOKER: Oh, it's all yours; it's all yours. I knew it was all yours.

DR. THOMPSON: Alright.

DR. HOOKER: See, I had seen, I had seen some earlier stuff . . .

DR. THOMPSON: Right.

DR. HOOKER: But Issa's staff had to redact the personal information, and yours took the longest.

DR. THOMPSON: Yeah. Of course.

DR. HOOKER: So, I saw everything that you had; everything from the letter C to the letter Z . . .

DR. THOMPSON: [Affirmative response.]

DR. HOOKER: . . . is what they had. Now they are not releasing this . . .

DR. THOMPSON: Yeah.

DR. HOOKER: . . . to me. They are letting me see it . . .

DR. THOMPSON: Yep.

DR. HOOKER: . . . and transcribe it by hand.

DR. THOMPSON: Yep.

DR. HOOKER: So, I'm trying to work behind the scenes with their office and with Posey . . .

DR. THOMPSON: Yep.

DR. HOOKER: . . . to get them to release this. And there may be . . .

DR. THOMPSON: It would be so great; it would be so great if you could get them to release everything. I'm just telling you that because it would take me off the hook. Then everything would be off of me, because then the records would be public. And then I could discuss them more.

DR. HOOKER: Well, let me . . . I will let you know how that goes, because I . . . You know, the clearest legal pathway is if they release them.

DR. THOMPSON: Yep.

DR. HOOKER: And there are some, there are some issues; there are some procedural issues with whether a committee chair like Issa can release those files directly. But I've told them, and I've said, "Look. If you can release them to Posey, Posey doesn't have the same restrictions because he's not a committee chair." So, anyhow I'll keep on pursuing those avenues. There's got to be . . . I would not be surprised if you had, if you turned over twenty thousand pages worth of documents. Because I didn't get through; I didn't even touch them. I mean skimmed.

DR. THOMPSON: No, I'm telling you; I'm telling you. I did a hundred thousand pages, so . . . You know, when you say you went through that many I mean . . .

DR. HOOKER: Well, well, mine's a wag; I mean that's . . . I'm probably low-balling it. I know that there are some things I have seen that were not in the documents that were in Issa's office. So, that was a little interesting. So, obviously some things aren't making it through the filter. But . . .

DR. THOMPSON: Oh, absolutely; absolutely I'm sure that's true.

DR. HOOKER: Yeah. Yeah. But I wanted to go to Barile.

DR. THOMPSON: Ah, Barile, Jack Barile.

DR. HOOKER: Is it Barile? Is it Barile?

DR. THOMPSON: Yeah.

DR. HOOKER: I could never pronounce it right. Barile. Okay.

DR. THOMPSON: Speaking of . . . You know these are the type of things. Whether you want to think things are coincident or not, he actually was . . . I actually had coffee with him this afternoon.

DR. HOOKER: No way.

DR. THOMPSON: He was here in Hawaii. [UI].

DR. HOOKER: Oh great.

DR. THOMPSON: So anyways; he's a great guy; he's a real young guy. And a very new . . .

DR. HOOKER: [Affirmative response.]

DR. THOMPSON: Actually he's . . . He, when we did that thimerosal paper (2012), he was still in graduate school.

DR. HOOKER: Yeah. I bet he has a great tan.

DR. THOMPSON: He does; he look [UI] . . .

DR. HOOKER: I mean . . . I, well . . . I got to say that; I'm from California. So, um . . .

DR. THOMPSON: Great.

DR. HOOKER: So anyhow . . .

DR. THOMPSON: Yeah.

DR. HOOKER: What I saw was . . . I saw some of the original versions of the Barile manuscript.

DR. THOMPSON: Yep.

DR. HOOKER: And I'm going to read some excerpts from the original, if you don't, if you can humor me. And it said [*reading*], "In light of these findings, the researchers conclude that the greater exposure to thimerosal from vaccines is potentially associated with an increased risk for the presence of tics in boys between ages seven to ten."

DR. THOMPSON: Yep.

DR. HOOKER: And that—I don't think that made it into the final manuscript. I mean how did CDC react to that statement?

DR. THOMPSON: Well, did I tell you . . . Alright. Did I tell you the story about this paper?

DR. HOOKER: No.

DR. THOMPSON: Alright.

DR. HOOKER: Well, you told me that they hired the tics guy, that you got this guy from Rochester.

DR. THOMPSON: Okay.

DR. HOOKER: Yeah. Are you there?

DR. THOMPSON: Yeah.

DR. HOOKER: You're kind of breaking up; I'm sorry. Are you still there? Let me check my connection; it might be me. Hold on. No, I'm getting good connection. Can you hear me?

DR. THOMPSON: Yeah. I'm going to go outside, just to make sure I have the best connection. Just a second.

DR. HOOKER: Okay. Okay. No problem. Alrighty.

DR. THOMPSON: Okay. This paper was the longest paper in clearance I've ever had.

DR. HOOKER: Okay.

DR. THOMPSON: It was in clearance for a year, and there's a really interesting story about this. So, Gabe Kuperminc, one of the other authors on the paper . . .

DR. HOOKER: Right.

DR. THOMPSON: Gabe and I went to graduate school together.

DR. HOOKER: Oh, no way.

DR. THOMPSON: Yeah.

DR. HOOKER: He was John Barile's advisor, right?

DR. THOMPSON: Yes. So, Gabe and I knew each other, and Gabe said he had this great graduate student. I said, "Great! I want to talk with you guys about a study I want to do." And I said, "I promised you; this isn't going to be easy, but I promise you, it's going to be interesting."

DR. HOOKER: Right. Good.

DR. THOMPSON: So, I, you know, I told Jack that he was going to be first author; I said, "Because you guys are outside the CDC, we'll have more leverage, 'cause . . . You know, you will have fewer constraints than I will."

DR. HOOKER: Right.

DR. THOMPSON: And I actually said, "If it gets really crazy, I'm willing to drop off as the coauthor and let you guys just publish because this was the public youth dataset."

DR. HOOKER: Okay.

DR. THOMPSON: So, anyways, we did the whole thing; we wrote the manuscript; we initially had pretty strong wording, like what you're saying . . .

DR. HOOKER: Right.

DR. THOMPSON: . . . about the association. And then it sat in clearance for a year, and people just hammered away at the paper and watered it down more and more and more. So, you got the manuscript you ended up with, which is the published manuscript—not the published; you ended up with the final, cleared manuscript with just the most, you know, whitewashed discussion ever.

DR. HOOKER: Right.

DR. THOMPSON: And then we got those reviews, and we were just thrilled with the reviews. And we were like, "This is great. Now we can bring back in our original text."

DR. HOOKER: Right.

DR. THOMPSON: So . . . You can really . . .

DR. HOOKER: Again, I have one of the whitewashed comments. It said, [reading], "Despite the significant association between thimerosal exposure in early life and the presence of tics in boys age seven through ten years, we think that thimerosal is not a major causal agent for tic disorder for several reasons. First, the magnitude of the potential contribution from early thimerosal exposure in the present study is small." I, I didn't get that. I mean . . . I, I . . . Was that referring to the risk ratios or the odds ratios? Or? I wasn't sure.

Dr. Thompson: Well, I . . . Well, the . . . There's . . . For a linear regression model, I call them beta coefficients. So, the beta coefficients were . . . You know, I mean . . . I'll give you my perspective. Any effect you find for any analysis like this is going to be small.

Dr. Hooker: Okay.

Dr. Thompson: I really do believe any analysis like this if we found something, it's not going to explain the huge increase in, you know . . .

Dr. Hooker: Sure.

Dr. Thompson: . . . autism cases or things like that.

Dr. Hooker: Right. Right. No, I understand that.

Dr. Thompson: So, it, it . . . So, whatever we found could explain a percentage of it, but, um, you know, I'd have to see the actual draft you're looking at. So, are you reading a comment that one of the reviewers made? You know, I believe . . .

Dr. Hooker: No, this was, this was . . . I don't know if this was from the final paper or if it was from a severely revised manuscript that then went out to publication; I couldn't really tell.

Dr. Thompson: Yeah.

Dr. Hooker: And I haven't cross-referenced this with the final paper.

Dr. Thompson: Yeah. I can't remember off the top of my head. All I have to tell you is we prepared, wrote a pretty strong discussion when we sent it into clearance. I knew they would whitewash it, and then we got these wonderful reviews, which was, you know, it was like a reality check for me.

Dr. Hooker: Right. I've seen those reviews. I got those in documents from Posey actually, so . . . And, and it was good; I mean it was very . . . It was an eye-opener; I hope it was helpful.

Dr. Thompson: Oh, it was three independent opinions, right?

Dr. Hooker: Right.

DR. THOMPSON: Three people who had no vested interest in the outcome of it and to say, "Why aren't you talking about significant results in the paper?"

DR. HOOKER: Right. Right. It . . . And it goes on. If I can ask, I have a quote, I have an email from . . . This was to you, and it's not concerning the [published] Barile paper, but your original manuscript . . .

DR. THOMPSON: Right.

DR. HOOKER: . . . the [*pause*] 2007 paper. This is from Nancy Levine [PH], and . . .

DR. THOMPSON: Yeah.

DR. HOOKER: . . . she, she's looking and she says, [*reading*], "WT, I think this document still needs language clarifying that the tic finding, even though it's statistically significant and repeats a finding from previous studies, is something you would normally find in this population." Well, they're kids, but you know that's . . . I don't get that. "I'm also concerned about . . ."

DR. THOMPSON: And Nancy, you know Nancy Levine is not a scientist, so . . .

DR. HOOKER: Well, why is she saying this?

DR. THOMPSON: . . . that's even crazier; that's even crazier.

DR. HOOKER: My first question is who the hell is Nancy Levine?

DR. THOMPSON: She's not a scientist; she's like an admin person. She's ah . . . I actually . . . I'm just wondering if you're reading it right. I'm wondering if she might have forwarded someone's comment.

DR. HOOKER: Oh . . . So, okay. Oh . . .

DR. THOMPSON: It would be really surprising for her to make a comment like that, but she might have. But that's what I mean; these are the type of people . . . She's a policy person. I think she calls herself a policy person, but I can't remember. But I mean, she is, she knows nothing about science. That's all I'll say.

DR. HOOKER: Right. Right. Well, I was, I was pretty sure, because she referred to, [*reading*] "I'm also concerned about saying that this finding should be studied further." I thought that was a, that was a travesty. Of course it should be studied further.

DR. THOMPSON: Of course it should be; of course it should be.

DR. HOOKER: And I'm not sure, ah, we want to say this or do this, but I'll leave it up to you and Ed, and that's Ed Trevathan. Is that how you say his name?

DR. THOMPSON: Ed Trevathan, who was the center director at the time.

DR. HOOKER: Okay. Okay. So, okay.

[Over talking.]

DR. HOOKER: [UI] . . . center director, yeah.

DR. HOOKER: So, if indeed these were her words, she was way out on a limb, because she is not a scientist.

DR. THOMPSON: Completely.

DR. HOOKER: Okay. Okay. And, um, now on your 2007 paper, was it submitted to Journal of American Medical Association or did it just go directly to New England Journal of Medicine? I thought it had gone directly to New England Journal.

DR. THOMPSON: I thought it went straight to New England Journal, but it might have gone to JAMA first; I can't remember.

DR. HOOKER: Okay. Okay. I . . .

DR. THOMPSON: I think it went to New England . . . I mean we all think, we all think the New England Journal is a much better paper, so I mean a place to publish . . .

DR. HOOKER: Oh, yeah. Yeah. Okay.

DR. THOMPSON: So, I don't know . . .

DR. HOOKER: It was just a hint of something that I saw.

DR. THOMPSON: I mean we might have been talking about which journal to submit it to.

DR. HOOKER: Yeah. Yeah.

DR. THOMPSON: But I can find . . . That's not, that wouldn't be hard to find. I'm, no, I'm 90 . . . No, we sent it to New England Journal; we didn't send it to JAMA.

DR. HOOKER: Okay. Okay. Well, let me make a note here. Didn't . . . Okay. That's what I thought. It's a good paper; it got good reviews.

DR. THOMPSON: Yeah.

DR. HOOKER: And the, you know, the conclusion still stands. Now, I went back; I mean this whole thing . . . You know . . .

DR. THOMPSON: Which it kind of reminds, which reminds me, I want to talk to you about the Verstraeten paper after we talk about this, because I have something really interesting to say to you . . .

DR. HOOKER: Okay.

DR. THOMPSON: So, go on.

DR. HOOKER: Okay. That would be great, but I went back to Tozzi.

DR. THOMPSON: Yeah.

DR. HOOKER: Because it looked like—and this I know—Tozzi was rejected by New England Journal of Medicine first. And there was a whole . . .

DR. THOMPSON: Who was?

DR. HOOKER: The Tozzi, Alberto Tozzi's paper.

DR. THOMPSON: Oh, Tozzi; I thought you were saying Posey, the Congressman. I'm like, "What?"

DR. HOOKER: Oh, no, no, no. He's not a . . . Yeah.

DR. THOMPSON: I think they say, I think they call him Tozzi, yeah, Tozzi. Yeah. Tozzi, Alberto. Yeah.

DR. HOOKER: And, so . . .

DR. THOMPSON: Yeah, his [paper] got rejected by New England Journal and JAMA.

DR. HOOKER: Okay. I thought I saw something—it said JAMA as well. I'm going to write that down. But what I did, I went ahead and I looked at his results for tics.

DR. THOMPSON: Yeah.

DR. HOOKER: And we've talked about this before.

DR. THOMPSON: Yeah.

DR. HOOKER: And so I just did a really simple student's T-test . . .

DR. THOMPSON: Yeah.

DR. HOOKER: . . . because we have the mean, the standard deviation, and the number [UI] . . .

[Over talking.]

DR. THOMPSON: Exactly, exactly. Exactly.

DR. HOOKER: They're statistically different.

DR. THOMPSON: I know. I know. I'm telling you. That's why I wanted you to look at it.

DR. HOOKER: Motor tics and phonic tics. Thank you so much, because they are statistically . . .

DR. THOMPSON: I know. I know, I know, I know.

DR. HOOKER: . . . completely different.

DR. THOMPSON: I know. I know. I know. But the . . . This is . . .

DR. HOOKER: The only thing that's odd . . . I'm sorry; go ahead.

DR. THOMPSON: But they, it really wasn't analyzed correctly, but I never went and did what you did. But I was looking at it, and I was like—I wish I had done it, but I wanted you to look at it, because I thought those raw numbers would be statistically significant. Just the numbers right in that table, so you confirmed . . .

DR. HOOKER: Yeah.

DR. THOMPSON: . . . what I thought. Yeah. Okay.

BRIAN: It was, it was . . . I haven't done males and females segregated yet . . .

DR. THOMPSON: Yep.

DR. HOOKER: . . . um, but overall, overall there is a statistically difference both in motor and phonic tics for . . . And so, so it confirms . . .

DR. THOMPSON: But that's why you got, you got to get the raw data. You can get the raw data if you guys put pressure on these guys. So, anyway . . .

DR. HOOKER: Okay.

DR. THOMPSON: Okay. And she can help; Nancy Levine was poking her head around trying to find out where the Italian data was; they were trying to find it and see if they could get it, but . . .

DR. HOOKER: Oh, wow. Okay. Well, I'll keep on . . .

DR. THOMPSON: Yeah. So, Nancy Levine is this policy person, and when you started requesting the dataset, I sent an email to Frank DeStefano and said, "Why don't we get the Italy data. That would be great to have, because X, Y, and Z." And he had replied back he didn't think we could get it. So . . .

DR. HOOKER: How did, how did . . . With David Shay . . .

DR. THOMPSON: Yep.

DR. HOOKER: . . . I saw an email between you and him . . .

DR. THOMPSON: Yep.

DR. HOOKER: It said, "Hey, sorry to bother you. I'm trying to pull together everything I sent to Alberto, et al. You don't want to know why." So, that piqued my interest.

DR. THOMPSON: Yep.

DR. HOOKER: "Can you recall when you sent me and can you find your original edits to the thimerosal draft we got from Alberto [UI] December, early January of this year." What was . . . Was . . . Where . . . They were funded by CDC, right?

DR. THOMPSON: Yeah. Completely.

DR. HOOKER: Okay. Who was the project manager on that? Was there a project . . .? Did they have project oversight . . .

DR. THOMPSON: Yeah. Yeah. Yeah.

DR. HOOKER: . . . or was it just a class or . . .

DR. THOMPSON: Yeah. Yeah. Yeah. Well, so, this is where you just got to understand the transition. So, David Shay was the project officer.

DR. HOOKER: Okay.

DR. THOMPSON: I was really the person who was doing all the work because I designed the [UI], you know, the [UI] neurodevelopment study.

DR. HOOKER: Right.

DR. THOMPSON: And we basically had Alberto do the exact same thing.

DR. HOOKER: [Affirmative response.]

DR. THOMPSON: So, we had Alberto take every instrument he could find and do it in Italian or whatever they wanted to do it in. And he basically replicated our design. So, I spent a lot of time with Alberto. Now David Shay is a pediatrician . . .

DR. HOOKER: Right.

DR. THOMPSON: . . . and, you know, he sat back and listened a lot.

DR. HOOKER: [Affirmative response.]

DR. THOMPSON: . . . and, ah, but he was technically the project officer. He was also the team lead at that point.

DR. HOOKER: Right.

DR. THOMPSON: Now, as I've told you, he resigned (from this project) in November of 2003 . . .

DR. HOOKER: Right.

DR. THOMPSON: . . . and went back to the Flu Division. And then he . . . I think he tried to stay on as the project officer, but Frank (Destefano) took over.

DR. HOOKER: Okay.

DR. THOMPSON: Now Frank is an Italian, and he owned property in Italy for a long time.

DR. HOOKER: Okay.

DR. THOMPSON: So, there was a long-term relationship with him and Alberto. So, anyway . . .

DR. HOOKER: With Tozzi. Okay.

DR. THOMPSON: . . . we, we funded the whole thing. They'll probably say . . . If you pushed it, they would probably say it was jointly funded.

DR. HOOKER: Sure.

DR. THOMPSON: But I believe the only grant money they had was from us.

DR. HOOKER: Okay.

DR. THOMPSON: Um, and here's the issue; understand my position. This was the best study of all of them is the first thing I want to say. Second it had a larger sample size than our New England Journal paper.

DR. HOOKER: [Affirmative response.]

DR. THOMPSON: Third there was true, true, true random assignment, and . . .

DR. HOOKER: [UI].

DR. THOMPSON: . . . and three it also found a language effect. So, it found the tic effect and the language effect. So, there were two effects that were replicated—I mean if you believe the tic effects were significant, which it blew my mind when the paper disappeared. The results disappeared for several years before I finally saw a draft.

DR. HOOKER: [Affirmative response.]

DR. THOMPSON: And that's why, I think that email that you saw was me like trying to figure out what happened to everything you saw originally.

DR. HOOKER: Oh, I see.

DR. THOMPSON: It was like, what the heck happened? How did it change so much? Because I was, I was really thrilled that it looked like we had something that had replicated. But, anyways . . .

DR. HOOKER: But it was very interesting because, and the reason why I keyed in on this, is then I saw . . .

DR. THOMPSON: Yep.

DR. HOOKER: I think it was a letter, I want to say it was from Melinda Wharton . . .

DR. THOMPSON: Yep.

DR. HOOKER: . . . or somebody in the ISO, and it was to a pediatrician who was very concerned about thimerosal and tics. And in this letter, she went on to say, "Oh well, we didn't see a consistent association in tics, because we did this Italian study by Tozzi et al., and they did not see an association with tics." And then, um, and then she was talking about speech delay and how there were several studies that you see a consistent association across the board. And once I did my analysis, I was like, "Bullshit. Come on."

DR. THOMPSON: Yeah. It's total bullshit. No, I know. But both of them, you have to realize . . . I worked with someone who worked closely . . . And I just have to tell you, I do not care for Larry Pickering.

DR. HOOKER: Sure.

DR. THOMPSON: Larry Pickering, I can tell you story after story about why that guy is, um . . . I don't want to disparage him, but I'll just say I don't think highly of him. But I had a go-between between Larry and I, and we went back and forth on what should go on the NVPO [National Vaccine Program Office] list of things to follow up on. And if you notice or know what that list is, it was tics and language delay. So those were the two things that went on . . .

DR. HOOKER: Oh, I . . . I saw that.

DR. THOMPSON: Yeah.

DR. HOOKER: Go. Go ahead.

DR. THOMPSON: So, yeah. So NVPO put it into what the CDC was supposed to follow up on, and the CDC never followed up on it. So it went into a National strategic plan for vaccine safety . . .

DR. HOOKER: Right.

DR. THOMPSON: . . . and that's what frustrated the hell out of me is they never did additional study after that.

DR. HOOKER: Right. Right. I did see . . . There was one thing I couldn't find the data on it. It was ISO's (Immunization Safety Office) response regarding recommendation nineteen for tics. And there was, you know, some odd number of . . .

DR. THOMPSON: Yep. Yep. Yep.

DR. HOOKER: . . . recommendations. [Reading] "Assessing whether thimerosal was associated with clinically important tics will be a research need for the ISO scientific agenda."

DR. THOMPSON: [Affirmative response.]

DR. HOOKER: [*Reading*] "ISO confers with NVAC (National Vaccine Advisory Office) . . ." Now they brought in NVAC's recommendations . . .

DR. THOMPSON: Yep.

DR. HOOKER: ". . . of a low-priority score." And, again, I just scratch my head. Like, well why would you? . . . I mean, this is the piece with thimerosal that is still left hanging.

DR. THOMPSON: Yeah, absolutely.

DR. HOOKER: So, um, that was very . . . So, so, NVP, and . . .

DR. THOMPSON: It was still . . . NVAC still had it on its list, alright? So it's on their list, but NVAC and ISO decide for themselves it's a low priority. So, you know, it's a very biased political agenda, you know, made it a low priority and, you know, created a situation that it would be difficult to get additional funding for.

DR. HOOKER: Do you think they would ever re-visit it? I mean, if we applied pressure and we started publicizing . . .

DR. THOMPSON: Oh, absolutely. Absolutely. No, no, no, absolutely. They absolutely would. And I do think you could do more studies. And, I've lots of ideas of studies you could do, so . . .

DR. HOOKER: Right, right. Because we want to apply pressure.

DR. THOMPSON: [Affirmative response.]

DR. HOOKER: And this is pressure that we could get somebody like Posey to appear at a press conference and talk specifically about this. I really want the Tozzi data. I'm, you know, you kind of inspired me to double my efforts in order to get . . .

DR. THOMPSON: Yeah.

DR. HOOKER: . . . that particular data, because I think it would be very, very useful. And in their analysis, they don't really, they don't really do any types of testing to show that their populations are different outside of mean plus or minus one standard deviation.

DR. THOMPSON: Yeah. And the other thing I was going to say to you about that analysis is, as opposed to the non-experimental studies where you need to adjust for things . . .

DR. HOOKER: Right.

DR. THOMPSON: . . . you actually shouldn't even, you don't even, you know, from a theoretical basis, you don't need to adjust for anything in that study.

DR. HOOKER: Right.

DR. THOMPSON: So, um, the second thing is, they had an unbelievable response rate. They had an 80 percent response rate from the original study.

DR. HOOKER: Wow.

DR. THOMPSON: It was like, it was like beyond . . . It was like your world's greatest dream. And the reason is, is because most kids in most of those villages don't move, so they're very easy to find.

DR. HOOKER: I'm going to call him. I might as well just . . . I have not tried that yet. I'll just call Alberto Tozzi directly. Explain.

DR. THOMPSON: Yep.

DR. HOOKER: You know, hopefully he, he won't think that I'm a demon like the rest of the CDC.

DR. THOMPSON: Yep.

DR. HOOKER: But, um, but I'm sure I can get his phone number. Um . . .

DR. THOMPSON: I'm sure you can get his phone number. You can at least email him.

DR. HOOKER: Oh, yeah. I've done that.

DR. THOMPSON: Okay.

DR. HOOKER: He, he does not respond to the emails. So, but I, you know, I'm not beyond stalking people. You know that.

DR. THOMPSON: Don't do it! Don't do it! Don't do it!

DR. HOOKER: No, not that way.

DR. THOMPSON: I would say, "Don't do it." No. No. I'm just saying that if he doesn't respond, you're not going to get him talking to you on the phone.

DR. HOOKER: Really? Okay.

DR. THOMPSON: Yeah.

DR. HOOKER: Well, I'll keep trying other avenues. So, now talk to me about Verstraeten. You were thinking, you were thinking about it.

DR. THOMPSON: Yes. So I was reviewing a paper that was doing a reanalysis of the Verstraeten study, and I re-read the Verstraeten article.

DR. HOOKER: [Affirmative response.]

DR. THOMPSON: And, um, I was actually talking to Chris Price about this this week who thought this was really interesting.

DR. HOOKER: Oh wow, okay.

DR. THOMPSON: So, if you have re-read the Verstraeten study lately, um, you will see, in the message section, that, um for Northern, for the big, I can't, I'm not supposed to say what HMO it is, but for the big HMO . . .

DR. HOOKER: Yeah. I know what you're talking about. Yeah.

DR. THOMPSON: . . . the one with 110,000 subjects, right? That's the one that had the tic effect, right?

DR. HOOKER: Right.

DR. THOMPSON: Right. And it's primarily because they had such a big sample size. So, the other HMOs had, I believe, positive effects, but they weren't statistically significant, right?

DR. HOOKER: That's correct. That's for both Harvard Pilgrim and the Group Health Northwest or whatever it was . . .

DR. THOMPSON: Right.

DR. HOOKER: . . . didn't have the effect.

DR. THOMPSON: Right. Right. So if you, um, if you looked at that, you would just say, "Well, they didn't have enough subjects when they did the other two, you know, when they used the other two HMOs."

DR. HOOKER: [Affirmative response.]

DR. THOMPSON: But, regardless, what's interesting to me is about other potential effects. And the reason I say that is, they have this sentence in there and I, I never really understood why they did it, but now I understand why it would significantly reduce the size of the effects. Okay? So if you look in the methods section . . .

DR. HOOKER: Okay.

DR. THOMPSON: . . . it says, "For NCK, we adjusted for which clinic the people were seen at." Because . . .

DR. HOOKER: That's right.

DR. THOMPSON: Because in some clinics they said there were higher rates of particular disorders. Now, and I think this is true at this particular HMO . . .

DR. HOOKER: Oh. Okay.

DR. THOMPSON: . . . but I'm not positive, okay? If, if the kids who have a . . . Like, if you test positive on a screener for any condition, and then that triggers something for you to be sent to one of the Kaiser specialists, right?

DR. HOOKER: Right.

DR. THOMPSON: So let's say you appear to have symptoms of autism, and then they said, "Well let's send him to the Autism clinic to see if he has autism." Right?

DR. HOOKER: [Affirmative response.] Right.

DR. THOMPSON: If you do that, then you would what you would do is essentially, are essentially creating a situation where some clinics look like they have higher autism rates than other clinics.

DR. HOOKER: [Affirmative response.]

DR. THOMPSON: And it could also be the case, for example, that if you are, if you, you know, if you live out sixty miles out of town, and the autism specialist is in town, right?

DR. HOOKER: [Affirmative response.]

DR. THOMPSON: You're going to drive in and go and see that person. So, if that's true and they adjust for that, they essentially adjust out any possibility for finding an association between the thimerosal and the effect. Because what they're basically doing is saying, "I'm going to co-vary out, um, co-vary out all the variation associated with neurodevelopmental outcomes from specialists."

DR. HOOKER: Right.

DR. THOMPSON: Where you would get the diagnosis from. I never really quite understood why they did that, and I was, I, I didn't have the data myself. I couldn't look at the data, but now I'm very suspicious about what that might do with some of the effects.

DR. HOOKER: That's a good point.

DR. THOMPSON: But I don't know. I guess you guys have access, you guys have access to that data so I might be overstating it. But it would be interesting to look at some of the other effects [UI] . . .

DR. HOOKER: Actually, I don't. I don't personally have the access. I requested a public use dataset for Verstraeten, and they told me to apply to the VSD [Vaccine Safety Datalink].

DR. THOMPSON: Yeah. You probably have to go into the, the . . .

DR. HOOKER: And in the VSD right now. See I tried to get around something through all the hoops that the Geiers jump through to get into the VSD . . .

DR. THOMPSON: Yep.

DR. HOOKER: . . . um, you know, because you had to go through all these different IRBs, you know, for each HMO that they were approved for and it was time-consuming and expensive. The Geiers are not approved to merge vaccine files. So you can't merge, you can't reconstruct Verstraeten, because you can't come up with the thimerosal dose.

DR. THOMPSON: Why?

DR. HOOKER: Um, they just, they . . . For some reason the way that they worded their proposal and Peter Meyer, you know, he's different. He may go for it. I might . . . I have nothing to lose by proposing a VSD study. I mean I really don't have any . . . The worst they could say is, "No," and I would just do a preliminary proposal and see where it went. And because the RVC is very, very different than it was in the early 2000s. It's a much friendlier place.

DR. THOMPSON: Yeah. When the Geiers went in there, there was no way they could manipulate the data appropriately just because of the constraints they were under. I mean . . .

DR. HOOKER: Well, and they didn't know SASS. They didn't know anything.

DR. THOMPSON: No, no, no. I know. But there were many reasons . . . That was a big mess both on the CDC end and then the Geier end.

DR. HOOKER: But it would be . . .

DR. THOMPSON: It went very poorly for everyone.

DR. HOOKER: Yeah. Oh yeah. Absolutely.

DR. THOMPSON: If you could get access to the data now and look at some of these things, my guess is they put that adjustment in there because they didn't like what they were finding.

DR. HOOKER: I would not doubt it.

DR. THOMPSON: And they only did it, they only did it for one HMO.

DR. HOOKER: They only . . . That's right. Oh, I remember reading that. That for the biggest HMO, they stratified based on clinic.

DR. THOMPSON: Yes.

DR. HOOKER: That is . . . Oh, wow. Wow, you hit the nail on the head.

DR. THOMPSON: Yeah.

DR. HOOKER: Um, and see, I always questioned that because I felt like you were matching out any variability in thimerosal, but I never really thought to question that out in terms of specialty clinics. In terms of specialists.

DR. THOMPSON: Yeah. If it was specialty clinics, then you're completely throwing off the associations because you're . . .

DR. HOOKER: Right.

DR. THOMPSON: . . . basically chucking out all the variants associated with the actual outcome.

DR. HOOKER: Right, right. You're comparing high with high, and high within high, and you can't do that so . . . That is really . . . I'm glad you caught that. That's pretty amazing. And it would be interesting to see what the tic outcome again would be, you know, if you could throw out those constraints for sure.

DR. THOMPSON: Yep.

DR. HOOKER: Okay. Alrighty. Thank you.

DR. THOMPSON: Yep.

DR. HOOKER: Um, I'm looking at my bucket list of questions. Okay, um, let's see. Talked about Nancy Levine; talked about David Shay. Um, the MMR paper.

DR. THOMPSON: Yeah.

DR. HOOKER: The, um, it looked like it was accepted in Pediatrics in July 2003 but it didn't come out until 2004. Is that pretty typical for Pediatrics? Does it take that long to get them . . .

DR. THOMPSON: I don't think it's that typical for it to take that long.

DR. HOOKER: Okay. I just thought maybe there was a story there or something. I don't know.

DR. THOMPSON: It's a story I don't know but you know, Pediatrics, JAMA, and New England Journal have very tight ties with the CDC, so . . .

DR. HOOKER: Yeah. It was very . . .

DR. THOMPSON: I don't know.

DR. HOOKER: I will tell you there was very sparse information.

DR. THOMPSON: You can do this. No. I know.

DR. HOOKER: Okay.

DR. THOMPSON: But you could do this. You could email Pediatrics and say, "What's the average time to publication when a journal's been accepted?" I think, just go look at some, go look at the journal Pediatrics, because they say when the article was received and then when it was published.

DR. HOOKER: Okay.

DR. THOMPSON: You can just go look. And go look at a couple of articles and see what the turnaround time is.

DR. HOOKER: Uh huh. I wasn't sure maybe if it was a peer review issue or, or . . . But yeah, I'll look. I'll look, for sure.

DR. THOMPSON: Yeah.

DR. HOOKER: Because there, there . . . It was very intriguing because there were . . . In your collection of information that went to Issa's office, there was precious little about the MMR. Everything with thimerosal, tics, thimerosal autism, the Price Study, Thompson Study, the Barile Study were all there. Nothing about what was there on DeStefano and so I found, I thought that was pretty interesting that there was . . .

DR. THOMPSON: Well, the DeStefano (2004 MMR paper) . . . Remember, I led all the analyses with the DeStefano thing.

DR. HOOKER: [Affirmative response.]

DR. THOMPSON: Literally everyone else got rid of all their documents so the only documents that exist right now from that study are mine.

DR. HOOKER: Right.

DR. THOMPSON: And it was the five of us. The reason you don't see anything else circulating on the study, it was five of us behind closed doors for two years.

DR. HOOKER: Wow.

DR. THOMPSON: So, that is why you don't see anything else.

DR. HOOKER: Right.

DR. THOMPSON: But what you do see, what you do see if you notice is . . . When I start getting pissed off that we're about to release some results internally.

DR. HOOKER: [Affirmative response.]

DR. THOMPSON: I don't know if those documents made . . . I think you've seen those; I've sent those to you. So, you know, in October of 2002, I was, you know, starting to share results and, um, that's when they reprimanded Bob Chen. Actually, it was early September 2002; I was ready to share results and I had notes that show we were going to even show them earlier and then, I do that early September and then, within two weeks, Bob Chen gets reprimanded.

DR. HOOKER: Wow.

DR. THOMPSON: And then several weeks later, we get FOIA; then we get legal people asking for all our documents . . .

DR. HOOKER: [Affirmative response.]

DR. THOMPSON: . . . and that's where there was the email exchange [UI] between Coleen Boyle and I about . . . You know, I was the only one that had documents. Everyone knew I was the only one that had documents. And I was like, you know . . .

DR. HOOKER: Right.

DR. THOMPSON: And that's when I considered, uh, you know, becoming a whistleblower, la de da di da.

DR. HOOKER: Right, right. Now, um, I did see that you proposed a thimerosal—Alzheimers study at some point.

DR. THOMPSON: Yes.

DR. HOOKER: Did, whatever happened to that? Did it just not fly?

DR. THOMPSON: Yeah. It just didn't fly. The other problem was just . . . The problem with that is, you wouldn't have any people exposed to thimerosal that would be old enough that you'd actually find cases of Alzheimers. So, you know, you have to realize the heavy doses of thimerosal came in the 1990s so, if you followed these people for fifty years, then you could do that.

DR. HOOKER: Right. Right. So the VSD would not be appropriate to study that.

DR. THOMPSON: Well, in fifty . . . I mean, you know . . .

DR. HOOKER: In that timeframe.

DR. THOMPSON: Yeah, 1995 plus fifty, which would be, you know, 2045, then you would.

DR. HOOKER: Wow. You're retired before then. Okay. Let's hope so.

DR. THOMPSON: I hope I'm still alive. I was going to say, "I hope I'm still alive."

DR. HOOKER: So, um, and then the . . . There were several documents that referred to what was called "Environmental Exposures in Autism." Was that . . . Is that just another name for the Price Study?

DR. THOMPSON: No.

DR. HOOKER: Okay. Because it looked like it was beyond thimerosal and so that's kind of what intrigued me.

DR. THOMPSON: Does it have, do you have a name affiliated with it? Because there's tables. We have lots of tables where we've described studies. So I'm just . . . If you can tell me . . . Anyway, the NIH . . .

DR. HOOKER: No.

DR. THOMPSON: Alright. There's one interesting study too. There's the NI . . . You and I have never talked about this study. There's a 2008 study that has Larry Pickering as an author.

DR. HOOKER: [Affirmative response.]

DR. THOMPSON: Where they went and did the biopsies. This Larry Pickering, Ian Lipkin . . .

DR. HOOKER: Oh yeah. I know all about this.

DR. THOMPSON: Okay. Did you and I talk about this study?

DR. HOOKER: Ah, no. You and I have never . . . I've talked to Ian Lipkin about it. In fact, he and I . . .

DR. THOMPSON: Okay.

DR. HOOKER: . . . are not speaking right now, because basically he doesn't like me very much. Okay?

DR. THOMPSON: Right. I mean, Ian Lipkin . . .

DR. HOOKER: [UI].

DR. THOMPSON: Right. Ian Lipkin is one of those . . . Well, I'll give you an example. When I was trying to hold them accountable . . . It was funded by the CDC.

DR. HOOKER: Right.

DR. THOMPSON: I don't know if you know that.

DR. HOOKER: Right. Right.

DR. THOMPSON: It was funded by the CDC; the money was sent to the NIH. It was the worst mismanaged event of federal funds that I've ever seen, um . . .

DR. HOOKER: Wow.

DR. THOMPSON: In terms of how that study was carried out. If you looked at the original study design and the fact that they only ended up with twenty-five Autism cases, it's just insane. So, I took over as project officer in the middle of that. And I kept trying to hold people accountable . . .

DR. HOOKER: [Affirmative response.]

DR. THOMPSON: . . . for what they were doing with the money and, um, the project officer on their end eventually dropped off the study; she was so fed up and tired with it.

DR. HOOKER: Okay.

DR. THOMPSON: In the middle, in the middle of the study, Ian Lipkin was asking for more money and he actually, and I . . .

DR. HOOKER: [Affirmative response.]

DR. THOMPSON: I don't think I kept the email but it's the one email I wish I had kept was where he said he was going to go talk to his Congressman if we didn't uh . . .

DR. HOOKER: [Affirmative response.] That sounds like Ian.

DR. THOMPSON: If we didn't give him more money.

DR. HOOKER: That sounds exactly like Ian Lipkin.

DR. THOMPSON: No. I . . .

DR. HOOKER: Oh my goodness.

DR. THOMPSON: No, he's an arrogant dick. And then the first author, Mady Hornig, I think she's first author on it.

DR. HOOKER: Yeah, yeah.

DR. THOMPSON: I'm not sure. So anyway. So Mady Hornig, who was doing animal studies, is his significant other. So . . .

DR. HOOKER: Right, right, right. They're shacking up.

DR. THOMPSON: So, you know, husband and wife team.

DR. HOOKER: They're shacking up. They're not married.

DR. THOMPSON: Yeah. Yeah.

DR. HOOKER: But, yeah. That's been historic. Yeah.

DR. THOMPSON: So, anyway. That was criminal because they published that study with twenty-five autism cases and the power was like zero . . .

DR. HOOKER: [Affirmative response.]

DR. THOMPSON: . . . and they tried to give the impression that they did a study of, you know, [UI].

DR. HOOKER: [Affirmative response.]

DR. THOMPSON: I don't remember exactly . . .

DR. HOOKER: They ran PCR in the cases. They ran PCR in the controls. They found measles virus in several of the cases, and they found measles virus in the controls and then they concluded there was no effect. But the actual conclusion of the study should be, "It's a really crappy study. We can't tell anything."

DR. THOMPSON: It was the worst study ever.

DR. HOOKER: Thank you.

DR. THOMPSON: It was the worst study ever.

DR. HOOKER: Thank you. When you talk to Ian Lipkin, he's like, "This is definitive. This shows there's no correlation."

DR. THOMPSON: It was the worst study ever.

DR. HOOKER: There's no such thing as autistic enterocolitis that has MMR . . .

DR. THOMPSON: It was the worst study ever. [Edited due to sensitive personal information.]

DR. HOOKER: Okay, okay. Well let me chew on this. You've given me a lot of assignments. I, I . . .

DR. THOMPSON: Okay.

DR. HOOKER: I love you and hate you for this but, um, but let me chew on this and, um, and I'll keep you in the loop in terms of the production we're getting from Issa and if we get anything from him so . . .

DR. THOMPSON: Well, we're going to give you an honorary degree in epidemiology, a Ph.D. in epidemiology if you follow through on these tasks.

DR. HOOKER: Bitchin'. You got it. Okay, okay. Alright. Hey, thanks a bunch WT.

DR. THOMPSON: Yep. Take care.

DR. HOOKER: Okay. We'll talk to you soon. Bye-bye.

DR. THOMPSON: Yeah.

Chapter 6
The Importance of the Thompson Transcripts

"There are only two mistakes one can make along the road to truth; not going all the way, and not starting."

—Buddha

It is difficult to overstate the importance of what Dr. Thompson, a CDC insider, says to Dr. Hooker about vaccine safety research. The bottom line is that he admits there are more questions than answers regarding vaccine safety. This should give all of us pause. We are told repeatedly by the CDC that vaccines are safe and effective. Yet someone whose job it is to test vaccine safety now says that simply is not the case.

This is critical information to Americans injured by vaccines who are largely without remedy from civil courts. Manufacturers of vaccines are protected from liability when their products cause harm. In 1986, Congress passed the National Childhood Vaccine Injury Act (NCVIA), which provided liability protection to vaccine manufacturers and health care providers. The vaccine schedule of the early 1980s was causing so many injuries and lawsuits that manufacturers threatened to stop making vaccines due an alleged lack of profitability.

DOSES of VACCINES for U.S. CHILDREN from BIRTH—6 YEARS

1983	2015
DTP (2 months)	*Influenza (Pregnancy)*
OPV (2 months)	*DTaP (Pregnancy)*
DTP (4 months)	Hep B (birth)
OPV (4 months)	Hep B (2 months)
DTP (6 months)	Rotavirus (2 months)
MMR (15 months)	DTaP (2 months)
DTP (18 months)	HIB (2 months)
OPV (18 months)	PCV (2 months)
DTP (48 months)	IPV (2 months)
OPV (48 months)	Rotavirus (4 months)
	DTaP (4 months)
	HIB (4 months)
	PCV (4 months)
	IPV (4 months)
	Hep B (6 months)
	Rotavirus (6 months)
	DTaP (6 months)
	HIB (6 months)
	PCV (6 months)
	IPV (6 months)
	Influenza (6 months)
	HIB (12 months)
	PCV (12 months)
	MMR (12 months)
	Varicella (12 months)
	Hep A (12 months)
	DTaP (18 months)
	Influenza (18 months)
	Hep A (18 months)
	Influenza (30 months)
	Influenza (42 months)
	DTaP (48 months)
	IPV (48 months)
	MMR (48 months)
	Varicella (48 months)
	Influenza (60 months)
	Influenza (72 months)

DTP- Diptheria, Tetanus, Pertussis (whole cell)
OPV- Oral Polio
MMR- Measles, Mumps, Rubella
Hep B- Hepatitis B
DTaP- Diptheria, Tetanus, Pertussis (acellular)
HIB- Haemophilus Influenzae Type B
PCV- Pneumococcal
1PV- Inactivated Polio
Varicella-Chicken Pox

Source: http://solospark.com/wp-content/uploads/2015/04/vaccines.
1983VScurrent.jpg

The 1983 immunization schedule for children up to age of six recommended ten injections of three vaccines (DTP, Oral Polio, DTP, Oral Polio, DTP, MMR, DTP, Oral Polio, DTP, Oral Polio).

Prior to vaccine manufacturers receiving liability protection in 1986, autism prevalence was 1 in 10,000 in the United States.

The CDC 2015 immunization schedule for children by the age of six recommends thirty-seven injections of ten vaccines. (Hep B, Hep B, Rotavirus, DTaP, Hib, PCV, IPV, Flu, Rotavirus, DTaP, Hib, PCV, IPV, Rotavirus, DTaP, Hib, PCV, IPV, Flu, MMR, Varicella, Hep A, Hep B, DTaP, Hib, PCV, Flu, Hep A, DTaP, IPV, Flu, Flu, Flu, Flu, Flu, MMR, Varicella).

In 2015, autism prevalence is 1 in 68 in the United States. The 1 in 68 figure is based on children born in 2002. In other words, the real rate may be much higher; we don't know.

Polio, MMR, DTaP were all on the schedule pre-1986. Hep B and Hib were added in the early 1990s at approximately the same time that the autism rate began to skyrocket. Chicken Pox (1996), Rotavirus (1998), Hep A (2000), PCV (2001), and Flu (2004) soon followed. (http://vec.chop.edu/service/vaccine-education-center/vaccine-schedule/history-of-vaccine-schedule.html)

If you are over the age of twenty-seven, you likely received the ten-injection vaccine schedule and you likely know very few peers with autism. If you are under age twenty, you likely received twenty to thirty-seven vaccines and you likely know many people with autism.

Autism prevalence is up more that 14,000 percent over the thirty-year period from 1985 to 2015. This increase eviscerates the theory that genes cause autism. There is no such thing as a genetic epidemic. The great autism gene hunt has been a failure. The dramatic increase of autism over the past twenty years must be attributable to something in the environment. Therefore, it is necessary to look for causative or contributing environmental factors. Based on tens of thousands of parental reports of children regressing into an autism diagnosis after vaccination, vaccines were a prime suspect.

The CDC and the Institute of Medicine went through a charade of investigating the vaccine schedule to see if vaccination had anything to do with the increase in autism. Rather than looking at all vaccines and the schedule as a whole, they purported to investigate ONE vaccine (MMR) and ONE vaccine component (thimerosal). Based on this superficial review, they declared in 2004 that the entire vaccine schedule was safe, and then thwarted additional research into vaccine safety going forward, as stated in the 2004 IOM Vaccine Safety Review.

Dr. William Thompson, a coauthor on MMR and thimerosal studies, now says the CDC has wasted ten years by failing to do credible research, even with respect to MMR and thimerosal—the only two aspects of the vaccine schedule that were looked at in the superficial review!

Parents, pediatricians, and policy makers have all been misled by the CDC and IOM. As Dr. Thompson says, "There are more questions than answers" regarding the effect of the vaccine schedule on autism.

If a coauthor of vaccine safety studies says there are more questions than answers regarding vaccine safety, how can states pass more vaccine mandates or restrict existing vaccine exemptions?

Other developed countries vaccinate much more cautiously than we do in the United States. Their citizens are not dying from infectious diseases. As opposed to the thirty-seven injections we have before age six, other developed countries give far fewer injections: Iceland (11), Sweden (11), Singapore (13), Japan (11, and pulled their MMR vaccine due to high injury rate), Norway (13), Hong Kong (13), Belgium (18), Austria (19), Israel (11), Denmark (12), Netherlands (20).

Many elected officials have no idea that so many vaccines have been added to the schedule. They simply don't realize that "having all your vaccines" means something very different if you were born after 1990. The next generation of American children need policy makers at all levels of government—federal, state, and local—to stand up to vaccine manufacturers.

In the past ten years, more children have regressed into autism. Their suffering could have been avoided. Lives and families have been ruined. A week does not pass without a report of a child with autism drowning, getting hit by a car, or being abused.

And what of those people in the medical and research community who have spoken out? What of those parents who asked questions about vaccine safety?

Those people have been marginalized, ostracized, and labeled "anti-vaccine."

For ten years, people in the CDC allowed this situation to continue and said nothing. They said nothing as children suffered, died and had their futures taken from them. They said nothing when others raised legitimate questions and often had their careers and reputations destroyed.

As Dr. Thompson states, no one has held the CDC accountable. That must change.

Chapter 7
Potential Next Steps
for Policy Makers

"Democracy is the worst form of government, except for all the others."

—Winston Churchill

Elected officials and policy makers at all levels should pay attention to Dr. Thompson's revelations in these transcripts and subpoena Dr. Thompson and his CDC coauthors to testify before Congress. It will be necessary to use subpoena power to require Dr. Thompson to testify because it is unlikely that his attorney, an expert in whistleblower cases, would allow him to testify unless compelled. Some of Dr. Thompson's coauthors told him that they would never voluntarily appear before Congress in the future. Congress would likely have to subpoena them as well.

Potential next steps for President Obama

- Support requests for a Congressional investigation regarding the 100,000 vaccine safety documents Dr. Thompson has already turned over to Congress.

- Assure Dr. Thompson of full protection under the federal whistleblower statute.

- Reassign Drs. Boyle, Yeargin-Allsopp, and Destefano to less sensitive positions—preferably positions unrelated to vaccine safety—inside the CDC while the investigation is pending.

- Realize that that the entire vaccine program is in the Executive Branch and hold the CDC accountable if the investigation proves Dr. Thompson's description of the culture of corruption inside the CDC is accurate.

- Request extradition of indicted fugitive vaccine researcher Dr. Poul Thorsen from Denmark to the United States to be tried for the serious crimes of which he has been accused.

- Immediately rescind the request for media censorship of vaccine safety issues, which apparently was authorized by the White House—and communicated by the HHS secretary—in 2010. (See Chapter 10.)

- Support the release of data, which the CDC collected for the Study to Explore Early Development (SEED) to an international independent body, such as the Cochrane Collaboration. The CDC and their partner organizations like Autism Speaks cannot be trusted to research this data honestly.

- Remove vaccine safety from the CDC's purview. The same agency cannot be responsible for promoting vaccine uptake and protecting vaccine safety. Dr. Thompson's suggestion of an FAA/NTSB model is reasonable.

- Support an Amendment to the Minamata Convention on Mercury, a U.N.-sponsored international treaty to limit environmental mercury exposures, to remove the exclusion for "vaccines containing Thimerosal" (Annex A, section E) as Thimerosal is known to cause tics and may be causing more severe harm.

- Issue an Executive Order removing Thimerosal from all vaccines in the United States as soon as possible because Thimerosal causes tics and may be causing greater harm.

- Support moving all vaccines worldwide to single-dose vials, eliminating the need for a toxic preservative. Work to improve cold chain storage in the developing world to make this possible.
- Support projects in the developing world for clean water and improved sanitation to combat infectious diseases. Supplement those projects with vaccination for diseases or conditions endemic in regions where clean water and good sanitation are not available.

Potential next steps for 2016 presidential candidates

- All of the above post-election if President Obama has not already done so.
- Oppose federal and state vaccine mandates because currently there are more questions than answers regarding vaccine safety.
- Support parental health choice and the universal right to prior, free, and informed consent to all medical procedures, including preventive ones.
- Realize that the current vaccine program is far different than the one you received as a child.
- Realize that the entire vaccine program is under the control of the Executive Branch. The next president needs to hold the CDC accountable on vaccine safety. Dr. Thompsons says, "Senior people [at CDC] just do completely unethical, vile things and no one holds them accountable."
- Rescind the request for media censorship of vaccine safety, which appears to be the policy of the Obama administration.

Governors

- Veto any bills increasing vaccine mandates.
- Veto any bills restricting vaccine exemptions.
- Governors are the last governmental line of defense between infants and vaccine manufacturers, which have full liability protection.

113

- Don't fall victim to media hysteria intended to scare people regarding outbreaks. Dr. Thompson describes how CDC and media "love" to "scare" people.

State Legislators
- Oppose any bills increasing vaccine mandates.
- Oppose any bills restricting vaccine exemptions.
- If your governor vetoes a bill, work to make sure the Legislature does not override the veto.

Parents

- Support Dr. Thompson for the courage it took to say what he did and encourage Dr. Thompson to keep talking.
- Work to make the transcript and audio recording of Dr. Thompson and Dr. Hooker go viral. Get it into the hands of other parents, your medical professionals, and any media willing to listen.
- Use social media, "alternative" news, health sites and blogs, and other non-traditional routes to spread this story. Past experience teaches that mainstream media is unlikely to touch this story due to pressure from their pharmaceutical advertisers and self-censorship. Censorship requests from cabinet Secretaries don't help. We likely need to bypass the mainstream media filters to reach our neighbors.
- Show this book to your pediatricians. Many will not like to hear it, but they were lied to by the CDC also. It's important for pediatricians to know that the safety studies they rely on every day when giving vaccines are not as honest and accurate as they may believe.
- Get involved in the political process and stay involved. If you are fortunate enough to live in a state that allows ballot initiatives, seek amendments to your state Constitution, which support free and informed consent and parental rights.

- Make sure that every 2016 presidential candidate knows about these transcripts and the culture of corruption inside the CDC that they describe.
- Thank Dr. Brian Hooker for making these recordings. Thank Barry Segal and his team at Focus for Health for making this information public.

Chapter 8
Conspiracy Theory or #1 Public Health Priority?

"It is difficult to get a man to understand something, when his salary depends upon his not understanding it!"

—Upton Sinclair

Why would the CDC rig vaccine safety studies, and how could they get away with it for fifteen years? Those involved in the corruption appear to be protecting three things:

1. **Protecting the vaccine program.** Protecting the vaccine program is one of the top public health priorities if not the #1 public health priority. The CDC personnel protecting the vaccine program are true believers in the "greater good" theory. And because of their unshakeable "vaccines save lives" belief, the CDC inflates the benefits and minimizes the risks of vaccination to benefit the greater good. The CDC rarely if ever mentions that the reason vaccines were given liability protection in 1986 is that they are by their nature "unavoidably unsafe" products.

2. **Protecting themselves.** For the past fifteen years, largely the same group of people has orchestrated vaccine safety research inside the CDC. Dr. Thompson names many of them on the four calls. This "inner circle" of CDC staffers has gotten away with rigging vaccine safety research for fifteen years because it is a small group. Dr. Thompson is the first to break ranks.

3. **Protecting vaccine manufacturers.** If the CDC staffers are interested in post-government careers, the natural place for them to work is the pharmaceutical industry. The most glaring example of this revolving door is Dr. Julie Gerberding, who was CDC Director during the period that the 2004 MMR paper Dr. Thompson discusses was completed. Merck manufactures the MMR vaccine. Dr. Gerberding left the CDC in 2009 and after one year (as required by law) joined Merck. Dr. Gerberding ran Merck's Vaccine Division from 2010–2014. Dr. Gerberding was promoted within Merck to Executive Vice President of Strategic Communications, Global Public Policy and Population Health at the end of 2014.

The corruption of vaccine safety research and the subsequent cover-up was also financially motivated. In the early 2000s, the CDC was under enormous financial pressure to cook the books to protect the vaccine program, the Vaccine Injury Compensation Program, their reputations, and their vaccine manufacturer partners.

Approximately four million children are born in the United States each year. Using the 2004 autism prevalence rate (1 in 166), that would mean approximately 24,000 total autism diagnoses per year at the 2004 rate. The 2009 award in the Hannah Poling case, a compensated case of vaccine-induced autism in the Vaccine Injury Compensation Program, was $20 million dollars.

Using the 2004 rate, and applying the Poling damage award, if 10 percent of the 24,000 autism diagnoses were caused by vaccines, the ANNUAL cost to the Vaccine Injury Compensation Program would have been ($20M x 2,400) $48 billion. If vaccines caused 20 percent, the ANNUAL cost would have been $96 billion.

Using 2014's 1 in 68 prevalence, there are at least 59,000 autism diagnoses per year. Using the 2014 autism rate and the Poling damage award, if 10 percent of the 59,000 autism diagnoses were caused by vaccines, the ANNUAL cost would have been ($20M x 5,900) $118 billion annually. If vaccines caused 20 percent, the ANNUAL cost would have been $236 billion.

(https://childhealthsafety.wordpress.com/2010/09/21/us20m-hannah-poling-vaccine-autism-case/)

In other words, over the past decade, the Vaccine Injury Compensation Program faced a potential $1 trillion obligation if vaccines were implicated in causing autism, or autism-like symptoms. The CDC had a trillion reasons to cook the books and find vaccines safe "on a population basis," as the IOM Committee was instructed to do in January 2001.

Chapter 9
Autism Speaks and the CDC Foundation

"In the end, we will remember not the words of our enemies, but the silence of our friends."

—Martin Luther King Jr.

Dr. Thompson spoke of the importance of the data collected through the SEED study. This data still is awaiting interpretation, which should be carried out by an independent body, such as the Cochrane Collaboration. Autism Speaks should not be part of any examination of that data, because it is too tightly aligned with the CDC and the pharmaceutical industry.

Home Depot co-founder and billionaire Bernie Marcus underwrote Autism Speaks in 2005 with a $25 million donation.

Mr. Marcus, a generous philanthropist, is a Board Chair Emeritus of the CDC Foundation. He was Chairman of the CDC Foundation from 1998–2001. Home Depot and the CDC are both headquartered in Atlanta. At the time of Autism Speaks' founding, Mr. Marcus also funded the Marcus Institute in Atlanta. Autism Speaks, the Marcus Institute, and the CDC have significant overlap in leadership.

One person who served on both the Marcus Institute board and the Autism Speaks scientific advisory board was Dr. Marshalyn-Yeargin Allsopp, a high-level CDC employee and one of the five coauthors on Dr. Thompson's 2004 MMR paper.

In a 2006 interview with *Investor's Business Daily*, Mr. Marcus demonstrated what may be interpreted as a pro-vaccine and pro-pharmaceutical industry bias when answering a question about being the CEO of a public company.

REPORTER: "Sounds like you're relieved to no longer be CEO of a public company."

MARCUS: "Absolutely. The worst thing I could imagine is to be the CEO of a pharmaceutical company today. I can't think of an industry that has done more to alleviate suffering and improve the human condition than pharmaceuticals. Yet the industry is under a withering assault from plaintiffs' lawyers and is depicted by some in the media as a pariah. I don't think that Jonas Salk could have developed the polio vaccine in today's legal environment." (http://www.legalreforminthenews.com/Reports/IBD%20Bernie%20Marcus%20Interview%201-30-06.pdf)

Based on Autism Speaks' long history of partnership with the CDC, and based on Autism Speaks' recent statement that "Vaccines do not cause autism," Autism Speaks cannot be considered an independent organization to be trusted to honestly research issues regarding vaccination using the SEED data going forward.

On February 5, 2015, Autism Speaks' Chief Science Officer Rob Ring definitively stated:

"Over the last two decades, extensive research has asked whether there is any link between childhood vaccinations and autism. The results of this research are clear: Vaccines do not cause autism."

Another reason to disqualify Autism Speaks as an independent organization for SEED data interpretation is its long history of hiring pharmaceutical executives. Chief Science Officer Rob Ring formerly worked at Pfizer and Wyeth. Before joining Autism Speaks, former Autism Speaks executive Peter Bell worked at Janssen Pharmaceuticals, the unit of Johnson & Johnson that manufactures Risperdal. (**Ring citation:** https://www.autismspeaks.org/about-us/press-releases/autism-speaks-names-robert-ring-new-position-vice-president-translational-re

Bell citation: www.autismspeaks.org/docs/d_200707_CNS.pdf)

When Dr. Thompson says he is part of the problem, and that the CDC set the research back ten years, please remember that Autism Speaks stood by the CDC's side throughout. Autism Speaks is also part of the problem.

Similarly, SAFEMINDS, an advocacy organization founded by Sallie Bernard, should not be considered an independent organization to study the SEED data, unless Ms. Bernard resigns her position on the Autism Speaks board. Ms. Bernard remained a part of Autism Speaks after their February 2015 definitive statement: "Vaccines do not cause autism."

Autism Speaks and its affiliates should not be entrusted to study the SEED data in the future.

Chapter 10
Media Censorship: Appeasing Advertisers, the White House, or Both?

"Our commitment to openness means more than simply informing the American people about how decisions are made. It means recognizing that government does not have all the answers, and that public officials need to draw on what citizens know. And that's why, as of today, I'm directing members of my administration to find new ways of tapping the knowledge and experience of ordinary Americans —scientists and civic leaders, educators and entrepreneurs—because the way to solve the problem of our time is—the way to solve the problems of our time, as one nation, is by involving the American people in shaping the policies that affect their lives."

President Obama, January 21, 2009
(https://www.whitehouse.gov/the-press-office/remarks-president-welcoming-senior-staff-and-cabinet-secretaries-white-house)

Has the federal government lived up to the transparency that President Obama called for in 2009? Or has there been tacit censorship on issues around vaccine safety?

Pharmaceutical companies are large advertisers in all forms of traditional media (television, magazines, and newspapers). Watch a national network evening newscast and count the pharma ads. Thumb through the Sunday *New York Times* one weekend and look at the ads. Look at any magazine and count the ads for drugs or personal care products.

Those who work for these media companies, their bosses, and their shareholders all know who their sponsors are. Without these advertisers, there would be even fewer media jobs. Basic business common sense would lead media companies to avoid stories that would upset their best customers if they possibly could.

In a May 2015 interview with Jesse Ventura, Robert F. Kennedy Jr. described a meeting with a senior television executive where the extraordinary influence of the pharmaceutical industry was highlighted.

"I ate breakfast last week with the president of a network news division and he told me that during non-election years, 70 percent of the advertising revenues for his news division come from pharmaceutical ads. And if you go on TV any night and watch the network news, you'll see they become just a vehicle for selling pharmaceuticals. He also told me that he would fire a host who brought onto his station a guest who lost him a pharmaceutical account."

Based on these considerations alone, the issues surrounding vaccine safety have had a difficult time getting a fair hearing in mainstream media. Frequently, the stories are one-sided.

Censorship was given White House backing when Health and Human Services Secretary Kathleen Sebelius stated the White House's policy in March 2010 in an interview with *Reader's Digest* while discussing the H1N1 flu.

"There are groups out there that insist that vaccines are responsible for a variety of problems despite all scientific evidence to the contrary. We have reached out to media outlets to try to get them to not give the views of these people equal weight in their reporting to what science has shown and continues to show about the safety of vaccines."

In August 2011, HDNet's news magazine defied the White House's censorship request and produced a story about how the federal government had indeed compensated cases of autism caused by vaccines in the Vaccine Injury Compensation Program (VICP). No one from HHS, the VICP, or the Department of Justice would appear on the broadcast to discuss these compensated cases. What happened to President Obama's support for transparency and open government? (http://www.ebcala.org/areas-of-law/vaccine-law/watch-hdnet-world-report-vaccines-autism-mixed-signals)

One of the few journalists to consistently stand up to censorship is Sharyl Attkisson, a five-time Emmy-winning investigative journalist formerly with *CBS News.* Ms. Attkisson recently published a book detailing her harrowing personal experiences as an investigative journalist, detailing efforts to stop her from reporting the truth and the decline of true investigative journalism. She now writes at her own website, sharylattkisson.com.

In February 2015, Ms. Attkisson posted an article on her website presenting her "Top 10 Astroturfers." Astroturfers are defined as "fake grassroots" organizations or individuals, where corporate or other special interests groups develop and use public relations budgets and non-profit organizations as a disguise—these AstroTurf organizations are really working on behalf of a special interests and not for the public. (http://sharylattkisson.com/top-10-astroturfers/)

Those who follow vaccine safety issues will recognize #3 and #4 on Ms. Attkisson's Top 10 list:

3. University of California Hastings Law Professor Dorit Rubenstein Reiss and Children's Hospital of Philadelphia's Dr. Paul
   Offit
4. "Science" Blogs such as: Skeptic.com, Skepchick.org, Science-
   blogs.com (Respectful Insolence), Popsci.com and SkepticalRap-
   tor.com

The websites and individuals Ms. Attkisson names are some of the
leaders of the pro-vaccine movement who try to portray themselves
as independent thinkers and independent organizations that are
independently funded, when they are not. Later in her article, Ms.
Attkission describes Asroturfer tactics:

*"Astroturfers often disguise themselves and publish blogs, write
letters to the editor, produce ads, start non-profits, establish Face-
book and Twitter accounts, edit Wikipedia pages or simply post
comments online to try to fool you into thinking an independent or
grassroots movement is speaking. They use their partners in blogs
and in the news media in an attempt to lend an air of legitimacy or
impartiality to their efforts.*

*Astroturf's biggest accomplishment is when it crosses over into
semi-trusted news organizations that unquestioningly cite or copy it.*

*The whole point of astroturf is to try to convince you there's
widespread support for or against an agenda when there's not.*

*The language of astroturfers and propagandists includes trade-
mark inflammatory terms such as: anti, nutty, quack, crank, pseu-
do-science, debunking, conspiracy theory, deniers and junk science.
Sometimes astroturfers claim to 'debunk myths' that aren't myths
at all. They declare debates over that aren't over. They claim that
'everybody agrees' when everyone doesn't agree. They aim to make
you think you're an outlier when you're not.*

*Astroturfers and propagandists tend to attack and controversial-
ize the news organizations, personalities and people surrounding an
issue rather than sticking to the facts. They try to censor and silence*

topics and speakers rather than engage them. And most of all, they reserve all their expressed skepticism for those who expose wrongdoing rather than the wrongdoers. In other words, instead of questioning authority, they question those who question authority. . . .

. . . A close third is an array of blogs that use words such as 'science' and 'skeptic' in their titles or propaganda in an attempt to portray an image of neutrality and logic when they are often fighting established science and serving pro-pharmaceutical industry agendas. These include: ScienceBlogs.com (using the pseudonym 'Orac'); vaccine inventor Dr. Paul Offit of The Children's Hospital of Philadelphia who earned an undisclosed fortune from Merck pharmaceuticals; and his apparent replacement in trolling blogs Dorit Rubenstein Reiss. She is a law professor at the University of California Hastings and a frequent contributor to SkepticalRaptors. com."

The AstroTurf organizations she mentions in her article, along with AstroTurf organizations like Autism Speaks, have been working daily since the news of recorded phone call first broke in August 2014 to keep the excerpts of Dr. Thompson's conversation with Dr. Hooker out of mainstream media. To date they have successfully kept the mainstream media from reporting this story. Now that the transcript has been released, we can expect these AstroTurf organizations to move into overdrive to keep Dr. Thompson from testifying before Congress.

We can hope that the release of the transcripts will change this dynamic, and mainstream media will report this important story.

At some point mainstream media journalists might, like Dr. Thompson, choose to listen to their consciences instead of their advertisers. It is time to report the truth: the vaccine schedule may be putting infants at unnecessary risk.

Chapter 11
First Principles and
Moral Courage

For Pediatricians:

"Primum non nocere (First do no harm)."

—Hippocratic Oath (circa 500 BC)

For Parents:

"Universal Declaration on Bioethics and Human Rights: Article 6—Consent

Any preventive, diagnostic and therapeutic medical intervention is only to be carried out with the prior, free and informed consent of the person concerned, based on adequate information. The consent should, where appropriate, be express and may be withdrawn by the person concerned at any time and for any reason without disadvantage or prejudice."

Adopted by the United Nations Educational, Scientific and Cultural Organization's (UNESCO) General Conference, October 2005

For Policy Makers:

"Few men are willing to brave the disapproval of their fellows, the censure of their colleagues, the wrath of their society. Moral courage is a rarer commodity than bravery in battle or great intelligence. Yet it is the one essential, vital quality for those who seek to change a world which yields most painfully to change."

—Robert F. Kennedy, 1966

If there are legitimate questions about safety of a medical intervention, the "first do no harm" founding principle of Western medicine and bioethics must be respected. With respect to vaccines, there undoubtedly are many unanswered questions concerning safety, as Dr. Thompson's statement on his attorney's website plainly shows.

Moreover, a first principle of human rights and bioethics regarding medical procedures is "free and informed consent." The Universal Declaration on Bioethics and Human Rights was adopted by representatives of 191 countries in October 2005. The language is crystal clear: "Any **preventative . . . medical intervention** is only to be carried out with the **prior, free, and informed consent of the person concerned.**" Prior, free, and informed consent to medical interventions, including vaccinations, is a basic human right.

If a state is going to force its judgment on a citizen or a parent regarding vaccination (a preventative medical intervention), the safety studies supporting those vaccines must be rock solid. According to Dr. Thompson, the studies are anything but rock solid. The quality of vaccine safety studies is insufficient to support mandatory vaccination.

Given what Dr. Thompson has disclosed, parents should not be removed from the decision-making regarding the health of their children. Parents know their own children's and their own family's health history better than their pediatricians and their elected representatives. Parents also know their religious beliefs and their personal relationships with God better than pediatricians, their elected representatives, and employees of their school districts.

No one is pro disease. The vast majority of Americans voluntarily receives most of the vaccines on the schedule. The relatively small number of people who vaccinate differently very likely have good reasons for making that decision. People who view vaccination differently should not be dismissed as "anti-vaccine."

The CDC, media, and vaccine manufacturers are good at scaring policy makers and parents. Consider that Dr. Thompson told Dr. Hooker—in May 2014—how the CDC and the media "loves" to "hype" measles outbreaks in order to "scare" the public. Dr. Thompson essentially predicted the hype and fear which surrounded the measles cases in early 2015 in California at Disneyland.

Where are the policy makers with moral courage?

Dr. Thompson wants to be compelled to testify before Congress with whistleblower protection. In order to testify as a whistleblower, with the legal protections that status invokes, Dr. Thompson needs a Congressional Committee Chairman to subpoena him. Similarly, his CDC colleagues should be subpoenaed to testify as well. Concerned parents nationwide need a Congressional Committee Chairman to conduct an honest investigation of the 100,000 documents he turned over to Congress. As Dr. Thompson tells Dr. Hooker, he anticipates that the four coauthors on his MMR paper will circle the wagons to try to isolate him. Fortunately, there are 100,000 documents in the hands of Congressional staff.

As Robert F. Kennedy said regarding moral courage, *"Few men are willing to brave the disapproval of their fellows, the censure of their colleagues, the wrath of their society."*

Which Committee Chairman has the moral courage to hold hearings on Dr. Thompson's revelations? There may be disapproval from certain donors. There may be censure from party bosses. There may be wrath from certain advertiser-supported media.

There will be push back from powerful lobbyists for the pharmaceutical industry.

But there may also be answers to why autism prevalence is up over 14,000 percent in one generation. It is also possible that the public will view the Committee Chairman who launches the hearings as possessing that rare commodity, moral courage.

In early to mid-2014, Dr. Thompson turned over the 100,000 pages to Congress. Yet, as of June 2015, approximately a year later, no hearings have been scheduled. As in the CDC, vaccine safety and autism is a scary political issue within Congress.

We can hope that governors will read these transcripts and act to protect informed consent. If there are more questions than answers regarding vaccine safety, then governors must veto increases in vaccine mandates and veto restrictions on vaccine exemptions until the safety issues are honestly addressed. If the CDC and Congress are both paralyzed because vaccines are "a political hot potato," then governors should err on the side of caution.

Hopefully, parents and organizations will spread the Thompson transcripts via social media. Perhaps increased attention to this story will help inspire Congress to convene hearings. Hopefully, some members of the mainstream media will also display moral courage and report honestly on this story. Few have been willing to do so to date.

Where are the editors and news directors who will report this story even if their corporate bosses disapprove? Where are the reporters who will ask President Obama if it is his policy to censor information regarding vaccine safety? Where are the reporters who will ask federal officials (and future presidential candidates) whether Dr. Thompson's role at CDC places him in a good position to have a credible opinion on vaccine safety? Where are the reporters who will ask President Obama if he thinks the United States should respect the Universal Declaration of Human Rights' standard of free and informed consent?

Who has the moral courage to be the modern Edward R. Murrow? What about moral courage in the scientific community? How do we avoid wasting more years on autism and vaccine research like the CDC and their partner organizations wasted the past decade? When Dr. Thompson said the CDC set the research ten years behind, he was talking in May 2014 and was referring back to the May 2004 Institute of Medicine report.

One important research project which has never been adequately investigated is a study comparing health outcomes in vaccinated populations with health outcomes in unvaccinated populations.

A pilot study comparing vaccinated vs. unvaccinated children has been done. Dr. Anthony R. Mawson, MA, DrPH (Doctor of Public Health), the principal investigator, is currently seeking publication of the results. Dr. Mawson is a social scientist and epidemiologist, and is a visiting professor in the School of Health Sciences, College of Public Service, Jackson State University in Mississippi. Dr. Mawson was also a professor of pediatrics and medicine at the University of Mississippi Medical Center, where he served as principal investigator of the National Children's Study for Mississippi.

Dr. Mawson's pilot study involves approximately seven hundred homeschooled children. The children in Mawson's study are arranged into three groups: fully vaccinated, partially vaccinated, and unvaccinated. Each of the three groups has roughly the same number of children. In general, the vaccinated population had significantly higher rate of chronic illnesses than the unvaccinated population. The vaccinated population had significantly higher rates of allergies, autism, ADHD, and learning disabilities. While Dr. Mawson's study is small, it does show interesting differences between vaccinated and unvaccinated groups.

Where is moral courage from the White House?

President Obama (or the next president if he does not act quickly enough) should clean house of all those who control federal autism research funding at the NIH and CDC. For years, projects like Dr. Mawson's vaccinated vs. unvaccinated study have been rejected as unethical, too difficult, or received a "low-priority score to disqualify it from funding."

As Dr. Thompson states, thimerosal causes tics and causes autism-like symptoms. It is abundantly clear that the CDC and the vaccine manufacturers will not remove the mercury-based preservative from vaccines unless they are forced to do so by regulators. It is time for a Presidential Executive Order removing mercury from all vaccines.

In 2014, the Autism CARES research bill was reauthorized through 2019 with no changes to the status quo. The agenda of the CDC and their Autism Speaks partners—which has set autism research ten years behind—remains unchanged. Most of the research funding goes to studies that avoid environmental causes of autism. If President Obama will not clean house at the NIH and CDC, then the next president should. It is time to move a genuine research agenda forward.

Where is moral courage in Statehouses?

The current vaccine system in the United States is not broken. Vaccination rates remain high. There is no need to increase mandates or restrict exemptions. The overwhelming majority of American children receive their vaccinations on schedule. Dr. Thompson's statements call vaccine safety research into question. The integrity of the CDC has been called into question. Dr. Thompson's revelations amount to research fraud and the CDC has betrayed the trust of the American people. Moral courage requires vetoes of vaccine mandates from governors.

Where is the moral courage from Autism Speaks?

The private sector autism organization with the largest research budget by far is Autism Speaks. Autism Speaks co-founder Bob

Wright knew about the audio recording of Dr. Thompson and Dr. Hooker's phone conversations as of August 2014. Six months later, on February 5, 2015, Autism Speaks released the following statement by their co-founder Bob Wright and their chief science officer Rob Ring:

"Over the last two decades, extensive research has asked whether there is any link between childhood vaccinations and autism. The results of this research are clear: Vaccines do not cause autism. We urge that all children be fully vaccinated."

—*Rob Ring, Chief Science Officer, Autism Speaks*

"Over the last two decades extensive research has asked whether there is any link between childhood vaccines and autism. Scientific research has not directly connected autism to vaccines. Vaccines are very important. Parents must make the decision whether to vaccinate their children. Efforts must be continually made to educate parents about vaccine safety. If parents decide not to vaccinate they must be aware of the consequences in their community and their local schools."

—*Bob Wright, Co-Founder, Autism Speaks*

(https://www.autismspeaks.org/science/policy-statements/information-about-vaccines-and-autism)

Autism Speaks claims to already know that vaccines are not related to autism, so they clearly cannot be trusted to research any aspect of vaccine safety.

The leadership of Autism Speaks is another example of the lack of moral courage. The grandson of the co-founders, Bob and Suzanne Wright, regressed into an autism diagnosis after a vaccine injury. Their daughter is very clear on this matter. Further, the Wrights have privately confirmed what they observed happen to their grandson yet remained silent.

Rather than risk the disapproval of their CDC partners, the censure of their billionaire underwriter or corporate donors, or the indignity of potentially being called "anti-vaxxers," Autism Speaks' leadership willfully ignored legitimate questions about vaccine issues for a decade.

Autism Speaks appears to believe they can only receive funding for other necessary work for autism in exchange for remaining silent on vaccine safety issues.

Autism Speaks cannot be considered an independent voice.

Congressman Bill Posey accurately described the failures of the federal autism research program in an op-ed article titled "Fix the Combating Autism Act," published in The Hill on June 13, 2014:

"Autism Spectrum Disorder has increased dramatically in the last 25 years. It is a crisis. What will legislators do with a federal program which, after eight years and $1.7 billion, has failed to truly address this crisis? Sadly, Washington is on a path to rush through a five-year reauthorization, raise spending 20 percent and hope for better results without addressing fundamental structural flaws in the current program. . . .

. . . At a recently called House Oversight Subcommittee meeting (May 2014), Dr. Insel admitted that after eight years and spending $1.7 billion, the programs developed in the CAA have failed to determine the causes of the enormous increase of the prevalence of autism, failed to prevent a single case of autism, failed to produce any new biomedical treatment for autism, failed to materially reduce the age of diagnosis of autism, failed to ensure appropriate medical care for the co-occurring health problems faced by many with autism, failed to ensure even basic safety protocols for people with autism who "wander," unfortunately some to their deaths, and overall, failed the families facing autism—most especially the approximately one-third of families with children most severely affected by autism, who literally cannot speak for themselves, and whose severe disabilities portend one of the largest unfunded federal fiscal liabilities of the 21st century."

(http://thehill.com/blogs/congress-blog/healthcare/209310-fix-the-combating-autism-act)

Chapter 12
What Needs to Be Done?

The White House, Congress, the press, and the American Academy of Pediatrics need to hold CDC accountable for the lies and deception regarding vaccine safety over the past fifteen years.

The White House

The entire vaccine program is under the Executive Branch. It's long past time for presidential leadership to take the issue of vaccine safety seriously.

If President Obama won't do it, then the next president must clean out the Immunization Safety Office and replace everyone but Dr. Thompson. Ideally, the replacements should do their best to resist unethical behavior, resist omitting significant data, and not lying in the first place.

Unfortunately, President Obama has done nothing to hold the CDC accountable on vaccine safety since taking office, so the task will likely fall to the next president. I truly hope I am wrong about the current president, but his policy appears to be tacit support for censoring vaccine safety issues.

Congress

Schedule hearings, issue subpoenas, and compel testimony under oath.

Dr. Thompson wants to be subpoenaed to be able to tell the truth. He no longer wishes to be part of a lie.

Where is the Chairperson of a House or Senate committee with the moral courage to call hearings and issue subpoenas? Which representative or senator wants to go down in history as the person who brought down the people responsible for the autism epidemic by shining a light on the corruption at CDC?

The Press

Where is the press on this scandal? Dr. Thompson is a coauthor of the safety studies the press cites, and he says he and his coauthors "deceived millions of taxpayers about the potential negative side effects of vaccines." Only one vaccine has ever been studied for safety regarding autism, the MMR vaccine. Dr. Thompson is a coauthor of the safety study, and he says he omitted data showing an elevated risk for autism from MMR vaccine in African American males. Only one vaccine ingredient has ever been studied for safety regarding autism: thimerosal. Dr. Thompson is a coauthor of the safety study which clearly shows that thimerosal causes tics. Thompson says that mercury-laden vaccines should never be given to pregnant women.

I understand that reporting on this story may upset pharmaceutical advertisers, but is it really a hard decision for news editors whether to cover a story which materially affects the health of infants? The CDC recommends that American infants receive six vaccines at two months old. After reading Dr. Thompson's discussion of corruption inside the CDC, and reading his admissions, how can this story be off limits?

The American Academy of Pediatrics

Pediatricians need to read what Dr. Thompson said to Dr. Hooker. Parents do not want to be in conflict with their doctors. Pediatricians vaccinated thousands of children due to fraudulent CDC science.

It is time for pediatricians to stand with parents and insist on holding the CDC responsible.

Governors and State Legislatures

The safety of the US vaccine program is now an open question. Until Congress completes an investigation of CDC corruption, it is irresponsible to increase vaccine mandates and restrict vaccine exemptions.

Parents may need governors to veto bills to protect their most vulnerable citizens. American families will remember those who acted responsibly at the polls.

Conclusion

"I was involved in deceiving millions of taxpayers regarding the potential negative side effects of vaccines. I regret what I did."

Dr. William Thompson email to Dr. Brian Hooker, August 11, 2014

William Thompson regrets what he did. When he sees a child with autism, he feels ashamed and understands that he should have come forward ten years ago.

What has happened in those ten years?

Our nation will soon have over one million people with autism. Thousands of children have been needlessly exposed to vaccines that were not as safe as they should have been. Families of these children struggle every day in ways that Americans who are unaffected by vaccine injuries never fully understand.

Like William Thompson, many parents who witnessed their children regress after vaccinations have been reluctant or unwilling to talk about what happened to their children. Many of these people know that they would encounter criticism, derision, and disdain from a country that has been oft re-assured that vaccines are always perfectly safe and effective.

Speak out? Why should anyone do that when all that awaits them is a label of anti-vaccine conspiracy theorist?

Because Dr. William Thompson was willing to tell Dr. Brian Hooker the truth, and Dr. Hooker recorded it, we now understand that the concerns of those often labeled "anti-vaccine" are completely legitimate.

The lies perpetrated by a small group of CDC employees have resulted in the nation's worst scandal since the Pentagon Papers. Daniel Ellsberg's groundbreaking journalism revealed that the Johnson Administration *systematically lied, not only to the public but also to Congress.*

The CDC Vaccine Safety Division has done the same here with fraudulent vaccine safety research. By omitting data, manipulating research, and lying to the public and Congress, the American people and Congress have been deceived. The pharmaceutical companies protected by these lies were only too happy to go along.

The human cost of this scandal is almost beyond comprehension. No amount of money, no amount of services, and no government action will ever undo the damage caused by this small group of CDC employees.

That doesn't mean that the damage should be accepted. As Dr. Thompson indicates, the lack of accountability must end. The White House, Congress, and the press need to hold CDC accountable for the lies and deception regarding vaccine safety over the past fifteen years. The same applies to the American Academy of Pediatrics—the nation's pediatricians have also been deceived.

This hands-off approach to the autism/vaccine issue, which every president has taken since the autism epidemic emerged in the early 1990s, is no longer acceptable. The Executive Branch is responsible for the Department of Health and Human Service, which runs the CDC. If President Obama won't take action, then the next president must reach down into the Immunization Safety Office and replace everyone but Dr. Thompson.

WHAT NEEDS TO BE DONE?

How corruption at the CDC caused the autism epidemic must now become a 2016 campaign issue.

If the Executive Branch won't act, then Congress needs the moral courage to hold hearings and subpoena those responsible.

State governments need to put the brakes on new vaccine mandates or restrictions on vaccine exemptions until independent science speaks on vaccine safety.

Dr. Thompson's statement that "there are still more questions than answers" regarding "understanding whether vaccines are associated with an increased risk of autism" is a bombshell. For years the mainstream press has lazily reprinted the CDC lie that science has concluded that there is no association between vaccines and autism, without reading the safety studies themselves. It is time for journalists to become *investigative journalists* again or else admit they are simply public relations firms for the pharmaceutical industry.

Science has been corrupted.

Pediatricians have administered thousands of drugs based on fraudulent science.

State governments are wrongly mandating more and more vaccines and removing parental rights.

The right to full and informed consent is being trampled.

Agencies that are supposed to protect public health have been captured by the pharmaceutical industry.

The Fourth Estate has been reduced to a PR firm.

Thousands of children have been injured and will need care for the rest of their lives.

There are painful lessons for our nation flowing from the words of Dr. William Thompson. Will we have the courage to reign in corporate influence over government agencies? Will we have the courage to admit that our government allowed a small group of people to injure hundreds of thousands of children? Will we have the moral courage to see to it that what William Thompson disclosed never happens again?

Author's Note

Before the end of 2015, please look for a recently formed organization called First Freedoms whose mission will be to ensure the next decade will not repeat the failures of the past decade.

If anyone would like to help First Freedoms in its mission, ideally on a scale similar to CDC Chairman Emeritus Bernie Marcus underwriting of the formation or Autism Speaks ($25 million), please contact me at firstfreedoms2015@gmail.com.

Acknowledgments

I would like to thank the people who made this book possible.

Thank you, Dr. Brian Hooker. Dr. Hooker's tireless effort directed at uncovering the truth regarding vaccine safety is by far the single most important factor in bringing the depth of corruption at the CDC to light. As readers can determine by reading the transcript, Dr. Hooker knows the flaws and is extraordinarily well versed in vaccine safety research. Clearly, Dr. Hooker earned the respect of Dr. Thompson, which is likely why Dr. Thompson chose to share this information with Dr. Hooker.

Thank you, Barry Segal, founder of the Focus for Health Foundation. Through this foundation and the Segal Family Foundation, Mr. Segal is committed to using the fortune he amassed through a lifetime of business success to leave the world in a better place than he found it. Without the structure Mr. Segal put in place, this book would not be possible.

Thank you, Dr. William Thompson. I would like to meet you someday to thank you in person. While listening to the audio recordings, your humanity and your genuine regret for your actions are evident. I hope Congress grants your request to be subpoenaed, so you can testify under oath to describe what happened inside the CDC. Thank you for keeping your records for the MMR study published in 2004, and thank you for turning over the documents to Congress.

Thank for apologizing to Dr. Hooker, and thank you for apologizing to Dr. Andrew Wakefield directly and through his wife Carmel.

Thank you, Dr. Andrew Wakefield. If Dr. Thompson and his coauthors had not rigged the data in their 2004 MMR study, Dr. Wakefield's scientific career would not have been ruined. Rather, Dr. Thompson says Dr. Wakefield's scientific opinion would have been supported. There were two extraordinary text exchanges between the Wakefields and Dr. Thompson in August 2014. (http://truthbarrier.com/2014/09/02/breaking-news-cdc-whistleblower-text-messages-to-andy-wakefield-study-would-have-supported-his-scientific-opinion/)

On August 20, 2014, Dr. Thompson texted the following message to Dr. Wakefield's wife:

"I do believe your husbands (sic) career was unjustly damaged and this study would have supported his scientific opinion. Hopefully I can help repair it."

That is one extraordinary text message. Dr. Thompson admits, ten years later, that if the CDC had not omitted data, the 2004 MMR study "would have supported his scientific opinion." Dr. Thompson watched for ten years while Dr. Wakefield was vilified, called a fraud, and had his professional career ruined. I hope all of those who have vilified Dr. Wakefield line up behind Dr. Thompson to apologize as soon as possible.

On August 27, 2014, one week after the apology text to his wife Carmel, and the same day Dr. Thompson's whistleblower lawyer statement was released, Dr. Wakefield had another text exchange with Dr. Thompson, which is arguably even more extraordinary that the first text.

Dr. Wakefield: Is the (Morgan Verkamp statement) press release real?

Dr. Thompson: Yes

Dr. Wakefield: Thank you. This was the right and honorable thing to do. Andy

Dr. Thompson: I agree. I apologize again for the price you paid for my dishonesty.

Dr. Wakefield: I forgive you completely and without any bitterness

Dr. Thompson: I know you mean it and I am grateful to know you more personally.

Dr. Andrew Wakefield is a hero for many reasons, including superhuman grace for forgiving Dr. Thompson. The sacrifices Dr. Wakefield has made and injustice he has faced are difficult to comprehend.

I'd like to thank the following people for their assistance in the production of this book.

Thank you, Tony Lyons, publisher at Skyhorse Publishing, for greenlighting this project. Tony's commitment to publishing books that shed light on the autism epidemic is second to none. If you are a parent of a child with autism, there is a good chance that the most helpful books you have on your shelf have been published by Skyhorse. Tony is an agent of change and he is doing all in his power to make quality information available through Skyhorse. He is an unsung hero.

Thank you, Lou Conte, consultant to Skyhorse Publishing, for assisting me at every step of the process. Your relentless good nature and your experience as an author were enormously helpful on a daily basis.

Thank you, Mary Holland, Kim Mack Rosenberg, and Rebecca Estepp, three of the most intelligent people I know, for helping me with edits on extremely short notice and the flimsy promise of drinks with cocktail umbrellas at some undetermined time in the future.

Thank you, Robert F. Kennedy, Jr. for writing the foreword. Parents of children who are vaccine injured and parents concerned about vaccine safety are grateful for your willingness to champion these issues. You are a true profile in courage.

Thank you, Dr. Boyd E. Haley for writing the preface. Your dedication to scientific integrity is admirable. If your warnings about vaccine safety have been taken more seriously a decade ago, it is likely American children would be more healthy. Thank you for all of your efforts.

Dr. Hooker, Dr. Wakefield, and Mr. Segal were not involved in the production of this book. Along with a few others, I was sent the transcripts of the four phone calls (and the audio recordings) in the hope that I could help bring public attention to this story. This book is a means toward that end.